This book is dedicated to my late grandmothers:
Rita Whitehouse and Mary Jane Tumminello.
From the day I was born until the day each of them passed on,
they spoiled me rotten and always made me feel as if their world revolved around me.
And that's the kind of love that every kid should grow up with and have in his life.

I'd also like to dedicate this book to my mother Faith Bevan
and to my father Dominic Tumminello. Although you both have very different outlooks
on life and on raising me, you both have done one thing that's exactly the same.
And that is not just being a wonderful and loving parent,
but also a best friend to me.

Strength Training
for Fat Loss

Nick Tumminello

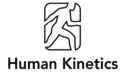

Human Kinetics

Library of Congress Cataloging-in-Publication Data

Tumminello, Nick.
  Strength training for fat loss / Nick Tumminello.
     pages cm
  Includes bibliographical references.
  1. Weight loss. 2. Reducing exercises. 3. Muscle strength. I. Title.
  RM222.2.T799 2014
  613.2'5--dc23
                                    2013042013
  ISBN-10: 1-4504-3207-7 (print)
  ISBN-13: 978-1-4504-3207-8 (print)

This publication is written and published to provide accurate and authoritative information relevant to the subject matter presented. It is published and sold with the understanding that the author and publisher are not engaged in rendering legal, medical, or other professional services by reason of their authorship or publication of this work. If medical or other expert assistance is required, the services of a competent professional person should be sought.

The web addresses cited in this text were current as of November 2013, unless otherwise noted.

Acquisitions Editor: Justin Klug; **Developmental Editor:** Laura Pulliam; **Assistant Editor:** Elizabeth Evans; **Copyeditor:** Alisha Jeddeloh; **Permissions Manager:** Martha Gullo; **Graphic Designer:** Fred Starbird; **Graphic Artist:** Kim McFarland; **Cover Designer:** Keith Blomberg; **Photograph (cover):** © Gary Rohman/age fotostock; **Photographs (interior):** © Human Kinetics; **Visual Production Assistant:** Joyce Brumfield; **Photo Production Manager:** Jason Allen; **Art Manager:** Kelly Hendren; **Associate Art Manager:** Alan L. Wilborn; **Illustrations:** © Human Kinetics; **Printer:** McNaughton & Gunn

We thank BB3 Training Center in Sunrise, Florida, for assistance in providing the location for the photo shoot for this book.

Human Kinetics books are available at special discounts for bulk purchase. Special editions or book excerpts can also be created to specification. For details, contact the Special Sales Manager at Human Kinetics.

Printed in the United States of America   10 9 8 7 6 5 4 3 2

The paper in this book is certified under a sustainable forestry program.

Human Kinetics
Website: www.HumanKinetics.com

United States: Human Kinetics
P.O. Box 5076
Champaign, IL 61825-5076
800-747-4457
e-mail: humank@hkusa.com

Canada: Human Kinetics
475 Devonshire Road Unit 100
Windsor, ON N8Y 2L5
800-465-7301 (in Canada only)
e-mail: info@hkcanada.com

Europe: Human Kinetics
107 Bradford Road
Stanningley
Leeds LS28 6AT, United Kingdom
+44 (0) 113 255 5665
e-mail: hk@hkeurope.com

Australia: Human Kinetics
57A Price Avenue
Lower Mitcham, South Australia 5062
08 8372 0999
e-mail: info@hkaustralia.com

New Zealand: Human Kinetics
P.O. Box 80
Torrens Park, South Australia 5062
0800 222 062
e-mail: info@hknewzealand.com

E5778

Contents

Acknowledgments

As I put together this list of acknowledgments, I'm taken on a trip down memory lane. And, that (memory) lane is a road that would not be paved to where it is if it weren't for the people on this list.

I have to start off by thanking my wonderful girlfriend, Jaclyn Gough, who is not only the sweetest and most beautiful person (inside and out) I've ever met, but she's that person we all need on our team who gives us unwavering love and support. I'm very lucky about a lot of things in my life, and one of those is getting to know you, Jackie, and grow closer to you more and more each day. Not to mention, Jackie is not only a big part of my life, but she's also a big part of this book, as she is one of the exercise models.

Big hugs go out to Deanna Avery and Paul Christopher for not only being some of the best friends I could ever ask for, but also for taking time away from their family and friends to model the exercises in this book. I also owe a debt of gratitude to Billy Beck (the Third) for his incredible hospitality in allowing us to do the photo shoot for this book at his facility: The BB3 Training Center. Each of you, Deanna, Paul, and Billy, are forever a part of this book, and I hope you're as proud to be a part of it as I am to have you as a part of it.

I have to give a shout out to my South Florida friends Rob Simonelli and Maggy and Alex Cambronero. The professional and personal support you've given me and Jackie is something you can't put a price on, and I'm forever grateful to call you our friends.

As an exercise enthusiast, I owe a big debt of gratitude to my longtime friend and fellow high school classmate Brad DeLauder. I could not have asked for a better weightlifting partner to share so much blood and sweat with from the time we were out of high school to our mid-20s. Those are some of the best memories I have, and I have Brad to thank for making that such a fun, memorable, and important time in my life.

I owe a special thanks to my mother, Faith Bevan, for not only being a great mom but for also raising me, as she says, "on the smell of iron and sweat." Going to the gym with you while you were training for your bodybuilding shows back in the '80s and seeing your dedication to leading a healthy and active lifestyle is clearly a big part of what made me who I am as a man and what I do as a professional. And to John Cavalier: thank you for being a great husband to my mother and a great friend to me.

If there is one thing that I have learned in life, it is that there are smart people and then there are good thinkers. Smart people are great at memorizing facts, but good thinkers are great at working things out. My father, Dominic Tumminello, not only taught me to always be myself—an independent-minded individual—but also how to be a good thinker to whom, as he says, "there are no problems, only solutions." This book is all about working out ways to use proven training principles to provide safe and effective training solutions. So, this book would not be possible if were not for the inspiration and life lessons I got from you, Dad.

As a professional fitness trainer, I owe a huge thanks to Marc Spataro, who is not only someone I love like a brother but the man who I was lucky enough to co-own a private training facility, FitNology (in Baltimore, MD), with for almost 10 years. I've always loved training clients and athletes, and working with Marc every day made it even better because I got to hang out with one of my best friends. This book would certainly not be possible if it weren't for Marc because all the techniques and applications featured here were developed and refined in the gym we co-owned together.

Firm handshakes and big hugs go out to all of my friends and colleagues who have taken the time to share their wisdom and experiences with me and who continue to help make me a better trainer and teacher and for making big contributions to the betterment of the fitness field: Bret Contreras, Brad Schoenfeld, Bob Esquerre, Jim Kielbaso, Mike T. Nelson, Jonathan Ross, Jonathan Fass, Alan Aragon, Leigh Peele, Mark Comerford, Bob and Ron Rossetti at North East Seminars, Shawn Myska, Rob Taylor, Vince McConnell, Mark Young, Bill Sonnemaker, Cassandra Forsythe, Jose Antonio, Roger Lawson, Mike Reinold, Eric Cressey, Tony Gentilcore, Ben Bruno, Dan Blewett, Yudi Kerbel, Dave Parise, Stephen Holt, Marie Spano, Jermey Shore, Mark McKean, Charles Staley, Ilene Bergelson, David Jack, Jon Erik Kawamoto, Luka Hocevar, Jonathan Goodman, and Claudia Micco.

I also owe a big thanks to my great friends and long-time clients with whom I got to spend a great deal of time with while I was in Baltimore: Mark Simon, Barbie Horneffer, Katie Horneffer, Sheila Fisher, Rufus Williams and Sheila Williams, Mary Hackney and Hap Hackney, Betsy Gorman (RIP), Moira Howen, Jeep Cochran, Maggy and Walter Brewster, Jen Watson, Kathryn Sweren, Alli Oliver, Henry Smith, Scott Anderson, Craig Rubenstein, John Rallo and the rest of the Ground Control crew, Binky Jones, Rick Desper, Elen and Charlie Rizzuto, Quinn Sypniewski, Kate Grevey Blankenship and Daniel Blankenship, Lindsay Janeway, Andrea and Larry Knight, Ken Wolf, Constance White, Lacey Morley, Annie Jenkins, Benji and Tim Jenkins, Morgan Johnson, Yoni Ronsenblatt, Gary Stastny, Nick Christo, Joy Blitz, Yudi Kerbel, Ellie Cox, Teri Rexroad Bickford, and Lisa Julio. Many of the names on this list are a big part of this book because many of the training concepts, techniques, and protocols featured here were first developed and used by them.

As a fitness writer, I must thank the Human Kinetics family—with special thanks to Justin Klug, Laura Pulliam, and Neil Bernstein—for allowing me the opportunity to share a piece of myself and the Performance University training concepts and techniques with the fitness world through this book. It's truly an honor to work with you and bring this project to life.

I've had the privilege of writing articles for many major fitness magazines and websites. None of those articles, or the writing experience and recognition I've gained, would be possible if it were not for Sean Hyson, T.C. Luoma, Lou Schuler, Bryan Krahn, Michal Kapral, Nate Green, Andrew Heffernan, Jen Sinkler, David Barr, Jim Casey, Alexander Zakrzewski, Jebadiah Roberts, Jerry Kindela, Andy Haley, Rachel Crocker, Jeff O'Connel, Nick Collias, Lisa Steuer, Lindsay Vastola, Adam Bornstein, Michael Easter, Greg Presto, Jessica Smith Gomez, Nick Bromberg, Erin McGee and Sarah Masi.

As a fitness educator, I have to send a big shout out to Benji Jenkins for helping me create my first 10 DVD projects, to Rio Santana for helping me put together my DVD projects to follow, and to Dane Davenport, who's done an awesome job helping me to continually develop the Performance University website (www.performanceu.net).

I also owe a big thanks to all of the professional fitness organizations and individuals who have given me the honor of presenting for them at their conferences, events, and fitness centers from China to Iceland and throughout the US. A special thanks goes out to the staff at IDEA and NSCA, along with Mike Bates and Nick Bromberg.

Last, but certainly not least, I owe a big debt of gratitude to Peter Bognanno and everyone at Reebok, to Matt Paulson and Hylete, and to Bert Sorin, Richard Sorin, and everyone at the Sorinex Equipment family, who have supported me over the years and provided me with the best fitness apparel and training equipment on the planet.

Introduction

Most books about fat loss are diet books. And, most diet books are based on fads that come and go like clothing styles. This book, however, isn't based on fads or miracle claims—it's based on scientifically founded training principles, sensible and realistic nutritional strategies, consistency, and hard work.

That's right—fat loss requires hard work and consistency. And that consistency involves not just how often you exercise but also the food choices you make. That being said, although what you eat is vital for fat loss, it does not take nearly an entire book to tell you what you need to know, nor does it require unrealistic, restrictive dieting. That's why this book dedicates one comprehensive chapter to nutrition—that's all you need—and focuses the rest on the exercise aspect of fat loss. Specifically, it explains how to use the three Cs of metabolic strength training—circuits, combinations, and complexes—to accelerate your metabolism and maximize fat loss while keeping muscle and even building muscle. Put simply, this book provides an easy-to-follow, realistic guide to ensure that the work you're putting in is as smart, safe, efficient, and effective as possible.

While the inexperienced exerciser will appreciate the simple way the information is presented, advanced exercisers and fitness professionals will certainly recognize the effectiveness or the principle-based training methods it presents and will gain exciting new ideas and organizational strategies for fat-loss training. So whether you're a beginner looking for a step-by-step guide to fat loss or a seasoned fitness professional simply looking for some new exercises to spice up your training, this book has more than enough for you!

This book is set up so that each chapter can be used as a stand-alone resource for training concepts and techniques that you can keep coming back to. In chapter 1, Benefits of Fat Loss, I present a number of reasons for losing fat that go far beyond just looking better. Sure, it's great to improve the way you look, but there are several health and performance reasons for losing fat.

In chapter 2, Strength Training and Fat Loss, I discuss the three Cs of metabolic strength training—complexes, combinations, and circuits—that are the basis of the exercise protocols in this book, describing what makes them effective methods for fat loss. In chapter 3, Nutrition for Fat Loss, I tell you everything you need to know (and nothing you don't) about how to eat in a simple, sensible and realistic way to stay healthy and accelerate your metabolism in order to maximize fat loss and keep your muscle.

In chapter 4, Circuits, I cover what a metabolic strength training circuit is, how to use the various types of fat-loss circuits, and how to perform a multitude of exercises using barbells, dumbbells, kettlebells, cables, and machines. In chapter 5, Combinations, I discuss metabolic strength training combinations and describe a multitude of combination exercise applications using barbells, dumbbells, and kettlebells. In chapter 6, Complexes, I explore metabolic strength training complexes and look at various complex exercise sequences using barbells, dumbbells, kettlebells, and Olympic weight plates. In chapter 7, Body-Weight Training, I show you how body-weight training can be used for fat loss by providing a variety of body-weight exercises, combinations, and complexes.

In chapter 8, Warm-Ups and Cool-Downs for Fat Loss, you'll get a variety of warm-up sequences and self-massage drills you can use to bookend your workouts and make your training well rounded. In chapter 9, Fat-Loss Workouts, I provide body-weight and gym-based beginner workout programs and intermediate workout programs to develop your training base. For when you've developed your training base or if you're an advanced exerciser, I also provide 6 months of metabolic strength training workouts that integrate a variety of circuits, complexes, and combinations into comprehensive training plans. Plus, I show you how to use the Fat-Loss Five workout protocol. And finally, in chapter 10, Fat-Loss Training for Life, I discuss rest and recovery, cross-training options, and the general rules of training safety and exercise selection to ensure you continue to achieve the best training results for a long time to come.

Now that you know what you're in for, let's talk shop!

Key to Muscles

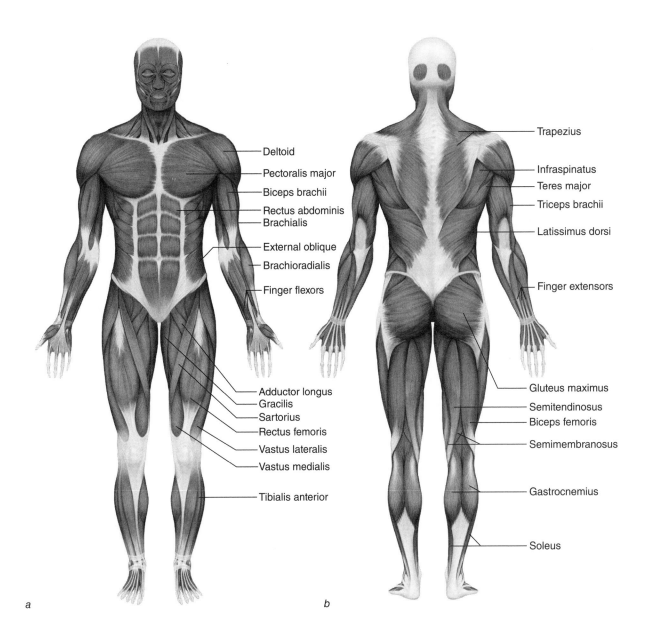

Deltoid
Pectoralis major
Biceps brachii
Rectus abdominis
Brachialis
External oblique
Brachioradialis
Finger flexors

Adductor longus
Gracilis
Sartorius
Rectus femoris
Vastus lateralis
Vastus medialis

Tibialis anterior

Trapezius

Infraspinatus
Teres major
Triceps brachii

Latissimus dorsi

Finger extensors

Gluteus maximus
Semitendinosus
Biceps femoris
Semimembranosus

Gastrocnemius

Soleus

a

b

Benefits of Fat Loss

Fat loss is almost always associated with appearance—just look at magazines, books, and TV infomercials for proof of that. It's no surprise, because a lean, athletic-looking body is something almost everybody wants. It helps us look better both in and out of our clothes. But, what about the improved health and performance benefits of losing fat and having a lean body? In this chapter I'm going to share the multitude of health and performance benefits that a fat-loss plan such as the one provided in this book can offer athletes, weekend warriors, and exercise enthusiasts.

BETTER SPORT PERFORMANCE

Two of the main performance criteria for athletes are how fast they can run and how high they can jump. That's why most coaches and scouts use some sort of jump test and sprint test for sports such as basketball and football. Now, most of us aren't making a living playing a sport, but we do enjoy playing sports with our buddies and family. Plus, it's nice to know you can move your body in the way you want to perform whatever activity you want.

Well, an effective fat-loss plan can help you run faster and jump higher! Imagine if you put on a backpack filled with 20 pounds of rocks and then sprinted 40 yards as fast as you could. Then you removed the backpack and ran the 40-yard sprint again. Do you think you'd run faster with or without the backpack? Of course you'd be faster without the backpack slowing you down because it's simply more weight for you to move. The same applies to jumping—it's obvious that you'd be able to jump much higher without the additional weight of the backpack.

That imaginary backpack represents the real-life performance limitations of carrying around an extra 5, 10, 20, or more pounds on your body. In other words, if you lose 5, 10, 20, or more pounds of body fat, it's like taking off a weighted backpack. When you lose the fat, you automatically become more athletic (run faster and jump higher). So, if you want to improve your sport performance, regardless of whether you're a weekend warrior or an elite athlete, an effective fat-loss program like the one in this book could be just the edge you need to outperform the competition.

IMPROVED STRENGTH

I just explained how losing fat can improve your hustle (i.e., athletic performance). Now, let's talk about how it can also improve your muscle.

One of the most important aspects of physical strength is what's commonly known as *relative strength*, which is how strong you are in relation to your own body weight. For instance, the person who can perform the most chin-ups possesses superior levels of relative strength because he can lift his own body weight for more reps than others can.

When performing strength training exercises such as push-ups, pull-ups, squats, lunges, and step-ups, you're not only lifting any free weights you may be holding, you're also lifting your own body weight. The more extra body weight you're carrying (i.e., body fat), the weaker you'll feel and the less work you'll be able to complete. Let's go back to our weighted-backpack analogy. Put on that weighted backpack and try to do squats, push-ups, lunges, and pull-ups. You'll do a lot fewer reps with the weighted pack on than without it. As another example, some people can't even do a single pull-up because they can't overcome their own body weight. Their training options in the gym become more limited, which can make their workouts less interesting and less effective. In short, the less excess body weight you're carrying around, the more weight and reps you can hammer out in the gym to continue to build muscle and increase strength.

BETTER CARDIO CONDITIONING

Extra weight won't only hold you back in the sport performance arena and in the weight room, it can also hinder your ability to play an entire game or go on a long hike with your friends and family. Cardiorespiratory conditioning is also known as *work capacity*, which is your ability to keep going before fatigue sets in. Regardless of whether you are playing a sport or going for a hike, you must have the energy to be able to go the distance. It's glaringly obvious that you'll get tired and quit faster when you're carrying around extra weight than you would if you had less additional body fat using up energy.

INCREASED ENERGY

We live in a world where we are inundated with energy drinks, most of which sell very well. It's beyond the scope of this book to get into the pros and cons of specific supplements such as energy drinks, but I can tell you that we all only have so much energy to spend each day before we feel fatigued.

As we've discussed, carrying around more body fat makes you work harder both in life and in sport. Therefore, the more extra body fat you've got, the quicker you'll get tired and feel the need for an energy boost. Carrying around that weighted backpack at your office or around your house will drag you down just as much as it does in the sporting arena or in the gym. Following a fat-loss plan will help you drop fat, which in turn will help you to become more energy efficient. This will not only make you feel better throughout the day, but you'll also save money because you won't have to keep buying those expensive energy drinks to get you through the day.

HEALTHIER JOINTS

Losing fat may help to minimize the risk of putting undue stress on your joints. You see, joints are avascular, which means they require regular movement (compression and distraction) to bring in nutrients and allow waste to leave our bodies. Put simply, our bodies respond to stress, and exercise and an active lifestyle can help us keep our joints healthy by giving them the movement they need. However, if you're carrying around extra weight, it can make you less comfortable with being active and, therefore, lead to a more sedentary lifestyle that isn't conducive to giving your joints the regular movement they need to stay healthy. Additionally, too much stress on our joints can cause them to break down and become less healthy. Considering the design and function of our joints, it is clear that carrying around excess body fat can turn otherwise-healthy activity and exercise into activity that overloads the joints beyond their capacity and place one at a higher risk of injury.

Furthermore, carrying around additional body fat can increase the risk of developing osteoporosis[1] and joint disease.[2]

HEALTHIER WEIGHT

In this day and age you don't have to be a cardiologist to know that carrying extra body fat (i.e., being overweight) can place more stress on your heart and put you at greater risk of dealing with health concerns such as diabetes, increased blood pressure, high cholesterol, and increased risk of heart attack. Maintaining a healthier weight by following the nutrition strategies and workout programs provided in this book can obviously lead to improved heart health, lower blood pressure, lower cholesterol, and lower risk of heart attack.

In other words, losing excess fat results in not just a body that looks good on the outside but one that is also healthier on the inside. Of course, certain genetic factors play a role in health concerns such as heart disease,[3] but that doesn't mean that we shouldn't do everything we can to minimize that risk.

LESS STRESS

Let's face it, we all want to look good, and there's nothing wrong with that. We have enough things to worry about in our lives, from work to finances to time management, that worrying about the way we look can be an additional stressor.

The good news is that not only can the workout and nutrition strategies in this book help you look better and feel more confident, they can also help you reduce stress in two other ways. One, they give you a user-friendly, easy-to-follow system that's based on sensible eating and fitness principles, not fads that will go out of style in a few years. This way you don't have to worry about the confusion created by conflicting information and constantly changing fitness and diet trends. This book gives you the simple, sensible, and scientifically-based direction you've been looking for. You just have to put in the work, which brings us to the second benefit:

The workout strategies in this book can help reduce stress because exercise is a great way to relieve stress. As you'll see as you get into the exercise chapters, this book provides more than enough exercises and workouts to keep you interested.

LESS ANXIETY AND DEPRESSION

Studies dating back to 1981 have concluded that not only can regular exercise improve mood in people with mild to moderate depression, but it also may play a supporting role in treating severe depression. Other research has even found that exercise's effects lasted longer than those of antidepressants.[4]

In regard to anxiety, research has shown that physical exercise reduces anxiety in humans by causing remodeling to takes place in the brains of people who work out. This evidence suggests that active people might be less susceptible to certain undesirable aspects of stress and anxiety than those of sedentary people.[5]

BETTER SLEEP

Sleep is the way our bodies rest and recover. And, in addition to elevating mood and reducing stress, research has documented the benefits of exercise to improving sleep patterns,[6] which can help you become more alert in the daytime and also help promote more sleepiness at night. Let's face it, if you're regularly exercising, especially using the programs in this book, your body will need to rest and recover, therefore making it more likely that your sleep will improve.

Now you can see why the value of a great fat-loss program goes far beyond just helping you look great in a swimsuit. It's one of the most valuable things you can do to improve the way you move in life, in the gym, and in sport and to keep you feeling healthy and reduce the risk of developing joint problems.

Strength Training and Fat Loss

Health and fitness can be viewed in three aspects: the mental, the physical, and the chemical. For any physical fitness program to be completely successful, especially one geared toward fat loss, it must be complemented by good nutrition (i.e., the chemical), and it must be something that you can get excited about and want to keep doing (i.e., the mental), because no program will work without consistency no matter how good it is.

This chapter covers the mental and the physical aspects. We're going to discuss not only why the workout concepts and techniques described in this book can improve your physical appearance and functional ability but also why they are more exciting than many traditional methods (such as cardio and bodybuilding training) and therefore may be just what you need to stay mentally engaged and look forward to every workout.

Muscle: Metabolically Active Tissue

Muscle is metabolically active tissue. In other words, muscle is the physical location in your body where stored body fat is burned (i.e., used as energy). More muscle requires more energy, so the more muscle you have, the more calories and fat you'll burn over a 24-hour period of time, even while you sleep! Although the exact number of calories burned for 1 pound (0.45 kg) of muscle is debated to be between 30-50 calories per pound, we can safely go on the low end of this: 30 calories burned per pound of muscle. That means that adding just 5 pounds (2.3kg) of lean tissue would result in losing one pound of fat every month—without any changes to your diet. And, a 10-pound (4.5kg) muscle gain would

effectively double the metabolic effect.[1] While a gain of 10 pounds of muscle seems like a huge deal to some people, the truth is that it's actually a trivial amount of muscle when spread over an entire body.

Put simply, humans are just like cars. If you put a bigger motor in your car (i.e., add muscle mass), you'll burn more fuel (i.e., calories) while driving (i.e., doing activities) than you did before. You want to be opposite of your car in that you want to become fuel *inefficient*, because the more fuel you can burn to perform a given activity, the better!

This is why strength training and maintaining muscle mass through proper training and eating strategies is critical for fat loss.

Put simply, you're about to discover why the *Strength Training for Fat Loss* training concepts and workouts are safe, super effective, and designed to be enjoyable enough to keep you coming back for more!

MUSCLE GAINS THROUGH STRENGTH TRAINING

Now that you understand why you need muscle to effectively burn fat, the questions then become "How do I gain muscle?" and "How do I keep (building) muscle while losing body fat?" It's no secret that the most effective method for gaining muscle is strength training. However, even fitness professionals seem to misunderstand the set and rep schemes that have been shown in the research to work best for increasing muscle (hypertrophy). You'll often hear people around the gym spouting off advice like, "Do low reps to bulk up and higher reps to get lean and toned." Unfortunately, that common advice is false. Here's why.

First, being "cut" as men often say and "toned" as women often say just means that you are lean which comes from fat loss. Second, most of the men seem to be comfortable with training to gain at least *some* muscle mass, but many women unfortunately think they'll get "bulky." This is just plain silly, since women have significantly less testosterone than men. So allow me to speak specifically to women for a moment.

When you talk about "toning," "enhancing," or "shaping" certain areas of your body, what you're really talking about is muscle. Put simply, muscle creates the shape of your body, and therefore more muscle equals more muscle tone. You can't build a perkier, rounder, or sexier *anything* without building muscle.

And, ladies: To build that muscle, you need to stimulate muscle tissue, and tiny dumbbells just aren't the tools for the job. Instead, women often benefit from the type of heavier lifting that they're more accustomed to seeing men do. Not to mention that, as I also stated earlier: Muscle is a metabolically active tissue, meaning it burns fat. Put simply, more muscle means a faster metabolism!

Third, your muscles don't become leaner by doing any kind of rep scheme, because muscles only have one way to develop: They either get bigger and stronger (hypertrophy) from strength training, or they get smaller and weaker (atrophy) from a lack of activity. Or, they stay the same. In other words, your muscles form the shape of your body, and being lean (having low body fat) simply allows you to better show off that shape.

Developing Your Muscle Base: The Foundation of Success

Building muscle is like building a house: They both begin with laying the foundation. For the metabolic strength training concepts and workouts in this book to be maximally effective and as safe as possible, you must first possess a strength training base. Developing a training base is the foundation that you build on, and the better your foundation, the more you can build on it. You wouldn't put on your shoes before you put on your socks. So follow the correct process—don't just skip ahead to the stuff that looks the most fun—and you'll get the best results possible. Spending 3 to 5 weeks developing a strength training base has several benefits:

- Strengthens your muscles, joints, ligaments, tendons, bones, and so on.

- Helps you become familiar with performing basic strength exercises using optimal form to prevent training-related injury.

- Improves your body awareness and the ability of your brain to better utilize your muscles. This is known as increasing neuromuscular coordination.

- Increases your metabolic engine by adding muscle. (Remember, muscle is metabolically active tissue, and more muscle means you burn more energy both while you train and while you sleep.)

Chapter 9, Fat-Loss Workouts, provides a workout plan for developing your training base if you don't already have one. Unless you're currently performing strength training a few times week, use the base training workout plan before starting the rest of the metabolic strength training workouts, also included in chapter 9.

Adjusting Sets and Reps for Muscle Gains

One of the keys to building muscle—to develop your base—is creating the stimulus to elicit muscle growth via the sets and reps you use. Different set and rep schemes have been shown to elicit different physiological and neurological responses. Here's an overview of the stimulus that each rep scheme creates.

One to 6 Reps

One to 6 reps per set are great for increasing muscle *strength* (i.e., force production) through primarily neurological factors such as increased motor unit recruitment. Additionally, this rep range serves as a nice middle ground for improvements in muscle strength and size. These rep ranges help your body bring more muscle into the game every time you use your muscles to lift a heavy load or explode in a sport event. If you think of your body as a computer, training in this rep range would be like upgrading your software so your computer runs programs (i.e., movements) faster and more efficiently.

Eight to 15 or More Reps

Eight to 15 or more reps per set have been shown to primarily stimulate increased muscle size (hypertrophy) through primarily physiological changes in muscles and connective tissues. Because this range uses a higher number of reps and lower loads, it creates more metabolic stress as well as an increased muscle pump, both of which have been shown to help increase muscle cross-sectional area (i.e., help you gain muscle). So, it's the higher rep ranges above 6 reps (8-15 reps) that are generally most effective at helping you gain muscle because it creates more of a physiological response. To go back to thinking of your body as a computer, this rep range helps to more-so upgrade your hardware.

The two set–rep schemes just described are not mutually exclusive. Mixing both schemes can have a positive effect—if you have strong connective tissues and bigger muscles, you can lift heavier loads (in the 1-6 rep range), and if you've become stronger and better able to use the muscle power you have, each rep you perform (in the 8-15 rep range) will be more effective than if you didn't have that improved neurological ability to recruit your muscles. Furthermore, although both rep ranges can facilitate positive improvements, you can certainly emphasize the rep range that best fits your goal. Additionally, a range of 6-8 reps can serve as a nice middle ground between the two rep ranges for improvements in muscle strength and size.

WHAT IS METABOLIC STRENGTH TRAINING?

The basis of this book is metabolic strength training, which means using innovative strength training concepts to accelerate metabolism in order to help you lose body fat while building and keeping muscle. In addition, the programs are designed to give you a great workout that you actually enjoy. Let's check out *what* the concepts of metabolic strength training are, *how* they work, and *why* they may be safer and more effective than other fat-loss training methods.

This book uses three metabolic strength training concepts, which I call the *three Cs* of strength training for fat loss:

1. Strength training circuits
2. Strength training complexes
3. Strength training combinations

Chapters 4 through 6 are each dedicated to one of the three Cs. In these chapters you'll learn what each of these metabolic protocols is and how to perform a multitude of practical exercise applications from basic to advanced levels using everything from barbells to dumbbells, kettlebells, medicine balls, stability balls, resistance bands, and cables. Additionally, chapter 7 covers body-weight training techniques using the three Cs, and chapter 9 explains the Fat-Loss Five circuit training formula. With all of the metabolic strength training concepts available in this book, you'll be able to immediately apply a large variety of techniques to help you incinerate body fat and dramatically improve your fitness and conditioning without losing muscle mass, regardless of your fitness level, space, or equipment limitations.

How the Three Cs Work

There are three reasons why the three Cs of metabolic strength training are extremely effective at burning fat.

1. *They're high intensity.*

   These workouts use challenging loads or lighter loads moved fast, both of which force you to work hard each time you move the weight. The higher the intensity, the greater the metabolic impact![2]

2. *They involve the entire body.*

   Each of the three Cs of metabolic strength training uses the entire body, involving your upper body, lower body, and core muscles. And, as stated before, muscle is metabolically active tissue, so the more muscles you work, the more calories you burn. The more calories you burn, the more productive your workouts will be—and the faster you will lose body fat.

3. *They demand extended repetitive effort.*

   Research consistently reports that a direct relationship exists between the duration of exercise and excess post-exercise oxygen consumption (EPOC), which is the number of calories expended (above resting values) after an exercise bout.[3] The metabolic strength training protocols in this book take more time to complete than a traditional strength training set. So, not only do they require you to perform high-intensity, total-body efforts, but you'll be performing them for extended bursts.

It's great to use scientifically proven workouts that have been evaluated in a study, but it's unrealistic to ask that of every workout, especially when we're changing workouts every few weeks to keep things fresh and interesting. Specific workout strategies don't have to be scientifically proven as long as they are scientifically founded, meaning they are founded on the general principles that have been repeatedly shown to elicit the results you're after. In this case, the three principles described in this chapter not only make scientific sense but also common sense. In other words, you don't have to be an exercise scientist to see how the combination of these three factors will burn a ton of calories and be super effective for losing fat and building metabolic muscle, something that a morning stroll on the treadmill simply can't match.

Furthermore, you'll find that the workout programs provided in chapter 9 don't just use one of three Cs for the entire workout. Instead, each program provides a comprehensive blend of the three to ensure each workout is more diverse and more effective. This is because, although founded on the same metabolic training principles, each of the three Cs offers unique benefits, and using all three more likely yields better results than exclusively using one.

Three Cs Versus Traditional Exercise Methods

We can't talk about new methods of fat loss like the three Cs without addressing traditional methods like cardio training, which is commonly thought of as the go-to exercise option for losing body fat. The first thing we're going to do in this section is give you the naked truth about cardio training by debunking some all-too-common, uninformed training myths. Then I'm going to provide a solid, common-sense rationale for why the metabolic strength training concepts in this book are a safer, more enjoyable, and much more effective training option for building the lean and muscular body you want.

Although any type of physical activity can have positive health benefits, the benefits of

Workout Intensity Is More Important Than Workout Duration

As I stated previously, workout duration is heavily linked to increased metabolic effects. However, doing longer workouts doesn't always mean that you're getting better results; in fact, it's likely that if you're just going longer, you're only able to do so because your overall workout intensity is less, therefore giving you the ability to last longer. Even in endurance sports such as triathlons and marathons, it's not about who goes the longest, it's about who finishes the fastest. In other words, it's about who has the most power endurance. With this reality in mind, you should progress in your training by continually trying to perform your workouts *better*, not just longer for the sake of going longer.

When you add sets or reps to your workouts, they will become longer, and that's okay.

However, you can't always keep adding on. You can also progress (make your workouts more challenging) by try to complete the same workout in less time than before, which boosts your working intensity. Or, you can try to get more work done (sets and reps or weight lifted in a given workout) in the same time frame that you did in the previous workout, which also increases intensity. As stated, there's nothing wrong with increasing your reps and working a little longer than you did previously, but solely relying on that method to progress is unrealistic and could lead to overuse injury.

Remember, you only have so much time in the day to work out. The goal is to get as much quality work done in that amount of time in order to maximize your results.

steady-state cardio training from a fat-loss (without muscle loss) perspective are often misunderstood and overstated. Especially because research has shown aerobic activity (cardio) to be the optimal mode of exercise—over resistance training—for reducing body fat in a timely fashion.[4] Now, these results are only half of the training puzzle because you don't just want a "lean" physique; you want a lean, strong and athletic-looking physique. And, in order to achieve the "strong and muscular" part, you've got to do resistance training, which is why the researchers of these types of studies also commonly state that a program including resistance training is needed for increasing lean muscle.

To understand why common statements such as "If you want to burn fat, do cardio" aren't very accurate, you must first have a clear understanding of what steady-state cardio training is and what it isn't. Once you understand what it is, you can better understand what it does and doesn't do for you.

You've probably heard the terms *aerobic training*, which means "with oxygen," and

anaerobic training, which means "without oxygen."

Cardio = aerobic training

Metabolic strength training = anaerobic training

The main thing that separates aerobic from anaerobic training is intensity. Here's a real-world example to help illustrate this concept: Let's say you and a friend are jogging together. While you are jogging, you are carrying on a conversation. If you're able to speak in normal sentences without any huffing and puffing between words, you're in an aerobic state. However, if you both decide to pick up the pace and speed up to a fast run or sprint, you'll still be able to talk to one another, but you'll be unable to get out full sentences without taking a breath, which means you're now in an anaerobic state. This example is called the *talk test*. It's a simple but legitimate method of telling whether you're in an aerobic or anaerobic state.

When you're in an *anaerobic* state, your body exclusively burns glycogen, which is what your body turns carbohydrate into after consumption. Glycogen is synthesized and stored mainly in the liver and the muscles. And, it's your body's preferred energy source. However, when you're in an *aerobic* state, your body has many options available to use as energy, including energy from glycogen, fat, and muscle tissue.

All of this information brings us back to the question, does aerobic training (i.e., steady-state cardio) exclusively use energy from fat? The answer is, no! Sure, steady-state cardio training can burn fat, but it'll likely use its preferred energy source: glycogen. And, it can burn from muscle tissue as well, which is why few endurance athletes have much muscle mass. Now, with physiology in mind, it's easy to see how cardio training sessions burn more overall calories than resistance training sessions. But, that fact is: it still doesn't mean that cardio is the long-term fat loss answer.

Sure, if you're looking for quick fat loss, I'd certainly say doing a few 20- to 30-minute cardio sessions per week is a good idea to get you quick gratification. And, it's unrealistic to think that doing some cardio for 4-6 weeks will turn you into a skinny endurance athlete with low muscle mass, especially if you're using them to complement a workout program that emphasizes strength-training exercise concepts such as the ones provided in this book. However, it does mean there's no need to go nuts and fall into the false belief that more cardio exercise means more fat loss—especially on a regular, long-term exercise basis. In fact, more cardio (with less or no strength training) will most likely lead to less muscle, which is not a good place to be in terms of strength, performance, or physical appearance.

Strength training is considered anaerobic training because it's high in intensity and burns energy exclusively from glycogen. That said, remember the previous illustration about talking while running together, and the faster you run, the more anaerobic you become? Well, the cool thing about anaerobic training is that it also gives you the benefits of aerobic training.

Think of a ladder: The higher you climb, the more intense the exercise becomes. In other words, the bottom rungs of the ladder represent aerobic activity, whereas the higher rungs of the ladder represent more intense, anaerobic activity.

When climbing up the ladder, you can't get to the higher rungs (i.e., anaerobic activity) until you've first climbed the lower ones (i.e., gone through aerobic activity). Additionally, when you climb down (i.e., recover) from the higher steps of the ladder, you return to an aerobic state. So, on both ends of anaerobic training intervals (i.e., sets of metabolic strength training) you also get an aerobic training effect. But, if you *only* do aerobic training (i.e., stay at the bottom of the ladder), you'll never get the unique metabolic and health benefits offered by anaerobic training.

The time between anaerobic bursts such as sprints or heavy lifting creates an aerobic effect while you allow your body to come down (i.e., rest) between sets. Again, high-intensity activities such as the three Cs of metabolic strength training have been shown to accelerate metabolism for up to 72 hours after the workout due to the effects of excess postexercise oxygen consumption (EPOC).[5] Steady-state cardio training, on the other hand, has not been shown to create nearly the same EPOC (exercise after-burn) effect.[6,7]

Each of the three Cs of the metabolic strength training featured in this book take anywhere from 60 seconds to several minutes of constant strength-based activity to complete. That's several minutes of high-intensity, total-body effort. Essentially, based on the scientifically-founded principles of fat loss, the metabolic strength training workouts get you better fat-loss results for your training time compared with traditional training methods.

WHAT MAKES METABOLIC STRENGTH TRAINING SO BENEFICIAL?

The human body has the amazing ability to adapt to the demands we place on it. As Aristotle said, you are what you repeatedly do. Earlier we talked about how becoming fuel inefficient (the opposite of your car) will help you burn body fat faster. What do think you're teaching your body to become better at when you train using lots of long, slow, distance cardio training? You're teaching it to become more fuel efficient because it knows it's got to keep as much fuel as possible to last for the long haul. In other words, due to the adaptive properties of the human body, doing lots of steady-state cardio training, on a regular basis for increasing distances, forces your body to become better at conserving energy (i.e., glycogen), which means you'll gradually burn less and less energy (i.e., calories and fat) as you become better trained. This is great if you're training to become a distance runner, but it's a problem when your goal is to maximize fat loss.

Metabolic Strength Training Versus Traditional Strength Training

If you're an athlete looking to improve your *conditioning*, which is the ability to resist fatigue during physical anaerobic activity, the training concepts and workouts in this book, especially the circuits and complexes, are just what the doctor ordered to help you outlast the competition. You see, traditional strength and power training methods are great for improving your peak strength and explosive power, but they're not so great for improving your *power endurance*, which is the capacity to produce the same level of power for a longer time—the length of competition. In other words, many of the low-rep, high-load training methods help you to peak your power in short bursts, but they don't prepare you to go five rounds or beat your opponent to the ball at the end of the fourth quarter.

However, training methods such as the complexes and circuits featured in this book do help increase your power endurance because they require you to perform a high amount of effort for extended periods of time, which is exactly what power endurance is. And, the principle of training specificity tells us that the adaptations to training will be specific to the demands the training puts on the body.

Metabolic Strength Training Versus Traditional Cardio Training

One pitfall of the false belief that steady-state cardio is the long-term answer to fat loss is the negative side effects of the two most common cardio training methods, jogging and cycling. Both of these training modalities are effective forms of exercise, and they're nice ways to get outside and do something active, but there are a few major drawbacks to doing them regularly. For example, both jogging and running (jogging is a slower run with a shorter stride) can be tough on your joints because for each step you take when running there is an impact force of about two to three times your body-weight. The impact force results from an abrupt decrease in velocity of the foot as it contracts the ground. And, in a 30-minute run, a typical runner will have about 5,000 impacts. So the accumulation of all those impacts that are likely the root of the injury problem. The impact force and the ensuing impulse wave have been identified as potential factors resulting in injuries, such as stress fractures, shin splints, cartilage breakdown, low back pain, and osteoarthritis, have been associated with these large forces and subsequent impulse wave.[8]

Also, most of us sit too much during the day. At work many of us sit at a desk, and at home we sit while using the computer and watching TV. It's no secret that sitting (i.e. being sedentary) isn't the best thing for functional capacity (i.e., our movement ability and athleticism), but physical activity is great for helping us to get lean and increase our strength and performance. Although cycling is physical activity, it is done from a prolonged sitting position where you're hunched over the bike. So, you're not only sitting all day at work and at home, but when you work out, you're sitting again! Plus, the cycling gets your body better at cycling, but it doesn't do much for strengthening your muscles for day-to-day activities.

This information is not intended to convince you to quit running or cycling, especially if you enjoy these activities. It's simply to inform you of their limitations and risks. That said, the workout programs in this book, which use the three Cs of metabolic strength training, provide a tremendous metabolic training effect without nearly the impact on your joints that comes from running or jogging. Additionally, the workout protocols are designed to fight the negative effects of sitting by training your muscles in more athletic postures and more dynamic movements.

If you do want to use traditional cardio activities, I recommend performing them at another time of day than the metabolic strength training program. For instance, you can do one type of workout in the morning and do the other in the afternoon. This strategy is especially helpful if you're using cardio on a short-term basis to get some quick fat loss, or for recreational activity. If you can't work out twice in the same day or prefer to get everything done in one workout, you can add cardio to the end of your strength training workouts because the cardio activity is less intense and less complex than the metabolic

strength training. But do not do cardio first because going into intense metabolic strength training in a semi-fatigued state will interfere with your performance.

The metabolic strength training concepts you're going to learn about in the chapters to follow are safer and more effective than traditional cardio training. Plus, they're more interesting and less monotonous than just doing the same activity at the same pace for an extended length of time.

As stated in the beginning of this chapter, for any physical fitness program to be successful, it must be complemented by good nutrition. As you know, the higher-quality fuel you put in your car, the healthier it stays and the better it performs. Unfortunately, the constantly changing diet fads and complex, often restrictive diet plans we are constantly bombarded with have left many frustrated and confused about a process that should not be much more complicated than putting quality fuel in your car.

chapter 3

Nutrition for Fat Loss

et's face it: What you eat and how you eat it can make or break the effectiveness of your program, regardless of how good it is. As the saying goes, although you can improve your fitness, you can't out-train a poor diet when it comes to fat loss (i.e., improving your physical appearance). In this chapter I'm going to share some simple-to-understand and easy-to-apply nutrition strategies to ensure that each meal you eat will help you accelerate your metabolism, more effectively burn fat, build muscle, and improve your overall health.

Knowledge is power. And, applied knowledge is empowering! I don't want you to follow the advice in this book just because Coach Nick says so. I want to help you to become an informed consumer. The goal of this chapter is to empower you with a solid rationale of not just what to eat but why to eat it. I also want you to understand that the nutritional information in this book is based solely on proven principles of the way the human body works—not based on opinions, diet fads, or unsubstantiated claims.

HOW THE BODY PROCESSES FOOD

As with exercise, there are some general principles for how the body processes food. Let's take a look.

Metabolism

Metabolism is the speed at which your body burns through the food you consume. Although we are stuck with our genetic makeup, we do have some control over the speed of our metabolism. Along with your age and gender, here are three factors that regulate metabolic rate:

1. *Activity Level*—This is how much and how often you perform physical activity.
2. *Thyroid function*—A calorie is a measure of heat, the body is a heat machine, and the thyroid regulates body temperature. Thus, it's obvious that thyroid function influences the speed of your metabolism. So those diagnosed with hypothyroidism can experience a slower metabolic function. The good news is this issue can be resolved through doctor-prescribed medication that works to normalize thyroid function.
3. *Body composition*—This is what your body weight is composed of, including muscle, fat, water, and so on. You obviously want a muscular physique, because, as we've established in the previous chapter, the more muscle you have, the more calories you burn over a 24-hour period, even while you sleep!

As you can see, two out of the three factors just described are things we have direct control over. If we follow an effective metabolic strength training program, such as those provided in this book, to increase activities levels and improve body composition—along with the nutritional strategies provided next—we can take control of our metabolism and accelerate it as fast as our genetic potential will allow.

Individuality

In addition to the three metabolism factors listed in the previous section, there are specific characteristics that can affect minor variables within your training program and eating choices. I'm referring to this as your *individuality*: It's what makes you different from the next person. Some of these variables include the following:

Metabolism

Genetics

Lifestyle

Stress levels

Profession (active versus sedentary)

Food preferences (what you like to eat)

Workout preferences

Even though we all are slightly different, we are made of the same raw materials, our bodies operate in much the same way, and thus the concepts in this book can work for everyone. Some of the minor specifics explained here as aspects of your individuality get worked out as you go along and discover more about yourself. Remember, you are the world's foremost expert on *your* body!

THE TRUTH ABOUT DIETS

When it comes to fat loss, most folks go on some sort of diet. Although it may seem like there is an endless variety of diets, the predominant amount can be classified in one of the following 4 types of diets:

1. Diets that cut calories
2. Diets that cut fat
3. Diets that cut carbohydrate
4. Diets that cut out certain types of foods

For the most part, I don't recommend any of them. Let me explain why.

Calorie-Restrictive Diets

Everyone knows the word *calorie*. Many people even know how many calories they are consuming per day. You may be one of them!

First, let's start with what a calorie is. Do you know? I'm always shocked at the number of people who talk about how many calories they eat, yet they don't actually know what a calorie is. A calorie is a unit of energy equal to the amount of heat needed to raise the temperature of 1 gram of water by 1 °C. In short, a calorie is a unit of heat, and the body is essentially a heat machine—hence the phrase, *burn calories*.

Now, before going any further, I want to make it clear that the relationship of how many calories you consume per day to the number you burn per day is the single most important factor when it comes to determining whether you lose fat. The concept that you need to be in a caloric deficit in order to lose fat isn't personal opinion nor is it up for debate by so-called diet gurus. This is the first law of thermodynamics, which states that energy can be neither created nor destroyed (conservation of energy), only changed from one form to another. And, this is validated in science as research looking into the potential advantages to diets emphasizing protein, fat, or carbohydrates have found that reduced-calorie diets result in clinically meaningful fat loss regardless of which macronutrients they emphasize.[1]

Although it's well-established that fat loss is determined by burning more calories each day than you consume, I'm still finding that most people don't need to bother with counting calories because if you follow the eating method I recommend, called *complementary meals*, you'll end up taking in fewer calories and burning more without ever actually counting calories, which is a pain in the you-know-what. I will explain complementary meals later in the chapter.

The main reason I'm not big on counting calories is the simple fact that not all calories are created equal. Some calories are more nutrient dense than others; we've all heard the term *empty calories* before.

Here's an example of why successfully losing body fat is not just about how many calories you consume. Let's say that we put two women of fairly equal size and fitness level on the same training program and allow them to eat 2,000 calories per day. Woman A can only get her calories from lean meat, fish, fresh fruits and vegetables, sweet potatoes, and rice. Woman B can only get her calories from candy, ice cream, and fast food. After 6 weeks, who do you think is going to look better, perform better, and feel better? Obviously woman A, because the calories she has been consuming are more nutrient dense and therefore contribute much more to her energy, strength, digestion, and so on. Both women may very well lose weight if they burned more calories each day than they consumed. But, woman A will still likely lose fat faster, keep more muscle, and have much better overall health because her fuel (food) kept her insulin levels more level and gave her more energy to fuel her activity. Let's face it—you don't have to be a nutrition expert to predict that even though both women trained the same way and ate the same number of calories, they will almost surely end up with different results. You understand this because it is easy to see how one can be well-fed but still not be well-nourished.

This is why when it comes to calories, my approach is to first emphasize the quality (i.e., nutrient density) of the foods you eat over the quantity (i.e., number of calories) and see where that gets you—it spells success for most people. It's certainly possible to eat too many calories from nutrient-dense, high-quality foods, so I will address counting calories later in this chapter as the second strategy to try after you've been using the meal formula described later in this chapter because, as I alluded to previously, when you concentrate on the *quality* of the calories you consume, you end up taking in fewer total calories anyway because most high-quality foods (e.g., chicken

breasts, veggies) are lower in calories. But, for those who've found their fat loss has plateaued or haven't seen much fat loss to begin with, counting calories is the next step needed.

Fat-Restrictive Diets

Put simply, too much fat in any form provides excess calories in the diet. However, simply cutting out all fat in your diet is not a good idea, either. Keep in mind that 1 gram of fat equals 9 calories, while 1 gram of protein or carbohydrate equals only 4 calories. So, if your current diet consists of 30 percent fat (or more) and you decide to simply cut it all out, you have just eliminated a significant portion of your overall calorie intake. If you drop your calories too low, you will drastically slow your metabolism and your body will likely start to feed off your muscle tissue for the energy it's no longer getting from the food you eat. In fact, most studies have found that the larger your caloric deficit, the more muscle you'll lose.[2-8]

When your body begins to feed off muscle tissue, it's called a *catabolic state*. This is not good because, as we've discussed, muscle is not only metabolically active tissue—the place where fat is burned—but it also is what gives you an athletic shape and keeps you strong.

Additionally, we all know how bad we feel when we don't eat enough and become malnourished. It becomes hard to concentrate on a simple conversation, much less perform well at work, hit it hard in the gym, or engage in sporting competitions.

Carbohydrate-Restrictive Diets

In the nutritional eating formula provided later in this chapter, I give some advice about minimizing your carbohydrate intake to maximize fat loss. That said, manipulating carbohydrate consumption and cutting it out altogether are two very different things.

To better understand why just cutting carbs is not the answer to fat loss, you must understand some basic facts about carbohydrates:

- The human body is fueled by glucose. All food must be converted into glucose before it can be used as fuel.

- Carbohydrate is more easily converted into glucose than protein or fat and is the body's preferred source of energy and the brain's essential source of energy.
- Glucose is stored in the blood, muscles, and liver as glycogen
- One gram of glycogen holds approximately 3 grams of water.

It's no wonder why people who cut carbs lose so much weight so fast—glycogen holds more than double its weight in water. It's therefore likely that they lost mostly water weight. This is why only using the scale to gauge your progress is a bad idea: The scale doesn't know the difference between muscle weight, water weight, and so on. In other words, there's weight loss and there's fat loss. When people say they want to lose weight, they mean they want to lose fat.

As you burn glycogen throughout the day, eating carbohydrate simply refuels your tank. If you suddenly stop refilling the tank, your body still needs a source of fuel for the brain, so it makes its own glycogen by breaking down muscle tissue and using it as energy. Again, this is a catabolic state, which is not good!

Food-Elimination Type Diets

In every fad diet there is always some specific enemy. In these diets, it is not a type of nutrient (fat, carbohydrate, etc.) that is the enemy, rather, it is a specific type of food or foods. Many of these diets take foods that a small portion of the population are allergic to, like foods containing gluten or dairy and advise everyone to avoid them as well, which is not only scientifically unjustifiable, it's like saying that since some people are allergic to dogs, no one should get a dog. Other diets demand that you eliminate a whole host of common foods that they claim are the "cause" of sickness and disease. Interestingly, these diets often make mutually incompatible claims as to which foods cause disease and which they claim to "prevent" disease.

In other words, some of the foods that are on the "no-no" list in one magic-bullet cure-all diet are emphasized as "good" to eat in another different magic-bullet diet. If this alone isn't enough to highlight why these "cure-all" type diets are based more on great marketing than they are on good science, keep in mind that every few years, there seems to be a new "cure-all" diet that claims to be better than the last. It's no wonder these diets never seem to gain any credibility among the legitimate medical and scientific community. Let's face it, if these diets worked as advertised, those who came up with them would get the Nobel prize and their methods would become standard practice in medicine and nutrition.

The fact is, what all of these elimination-type diets do is take an extreme approach to problems that can be solved with good old moderation. In short, unless you have a genuine food allergy—diagnosed by a real doctor—then there's no need for you to fully eliminate any type of food or ingredient from your diet. You just have to consume the foods that aren't so healthy in moderation. If there is an exception to this I'd say it would be to eliminate trans fats from partially hydrogenated oils, as even small amounts of trans fat in the diet can have harmful health effects. For every extra 2 percent of calories from trans fat daily, the risk of coronary heart disease increases by 23 percent.[9]

THE NO-DIET DIET SOLUTION

When all is said and done, the long-term solution is not to simply cut certain foods out of your diet but to replace what you're currently eating with better and more thermic foods that your body can use. This is what I call *complementary eating*. Complementary eating is a simple, practical, and realistic eating strategy you can use to ensure that each meal you eat will help you more effectively burn fat, build muscle, and improve your overall health.

What Is Complementary Eating?

A complementary meal consists of four components:

1. Protein (eggs, chicken, fish, bison, beef, and so on)
2. Fibrous carbohydrate (fruits and vegetables)
3. Starchy carbohydrate (sweet potatoes, rice, oatmeal, and so on)
4. Fat (avocado, nuts, olive oil, and so on)

We call this strategy *complementary eating* because each component of the meal complements the others to maximize nutritional benefits.

- Protein is the building block of muscle.
- Starchy carbs are a great energy source.
- Fibrous carbs move it all through the body and provide energy.

- Fat decreases inflammation, improves joint and heart health, and aids in disease prevention and cognitive function.

Additionally, complementary eating can help you emphasize fresh, local fruits and vegetables and high-quality meats, eggs, and fish while limiting processed food, simple sugar, hydrogenated oil, and alcohol. There's nothing wrong with having a glass of wine or a beer here and there when you're trying to lose fat. Just understand that alcohol is the simplest sugar there is.

Figure 3.1 is a list of recommended foods based on the idea of complementary eating. It is not an exhaustive list but just a few food choices to emphasize.

Figure 3.1 Recommended Foods for Complementary Eating

PROTEIN

Chicken breast
Turkey (tenderloin, breast, or ground lean white meat)
Salmon
Tilapia
Halibut
Tuna (fresh or canned)
Orange roughy
Shrimp
Bison
Lean ground beef
Lean cuts of red meat
Eggs
Pork

CONDIMENTS

Mustard
Hot Sauce

STARCHY CARBOHYDRATE

Brown or white rice
Jasmine rice
Oatmeal
Oat bran
Quinoa
Chia seeds (try putting them in shakes)
Sweet potatoes
Black beans
Rice cakes

FAT

Olive oil
Truffle oil
Fish oil
Peanut butter (natural) or almond butter
Avocado
Almonds and other nuts

VEGETABLES

Broccoli
Spinach
Asparagus
Peppers
Zucchini
Mushrooms
Green beans
Onions
Cucumbers
Fruits

FRUITS

Apricots
Blackberries
Figs
Grapefruit
Oranges
Papayas
Peaches
Plums
Raspberries
Strawberries
Blueberries
Tomatoes

With complementary eating, try to eat three to four meals per day. Meal size differs for everyone and should be based on how you feel and how much fuel your body requires that day. In general, size your complementary meal portions in this manner:

- Make the protein and fibrous veggies the largest portion on your plate. (Note: High-protein meals create a sense of fullness, which helps to reduce excessive caloric intake and promote fat loss.)
- Make the starchy carbohydrate and fruit smaller than the protein and veggies.
- Make the healthy fat the smallest serving on your plate.

If you feel hungry within an hour or so after finishing your meal, you probably didn't eat enough. On the flip side, if you feel full for hours, you probably ate too much. It comes down to common sense, intuition, and simply listening to your body. Also, the concept of eating five to six meals throughout the day is unrealistic for most people, and the evidence doesn't support this eating habit. Research has shown that those who ate six meals a day exhibited significantly higher blood sugar levels than those who ate three meals a day.[15] That means that eating fewer meals throughout the day allows your body to lower blood sugar levels more efficiently, create a physiological environment more conducive to fat loss.

How Does Complementary Eating Work?

As discussed previously, a calorie is a measure of heat, and your body is a heat machine. The term *thermic effect of food*, or TEF, is used to describe the energy expended by our bodies in order to consume (bite, chew, and swallow) and process (digest, transport, metabolize, and store) food. In other words, certain foods require us to burn more calories than others simply by eating them. Here's the general breakdown:

- *Fat* is easy to digest. Your body simply keeps breaking down the fat molecules smaller and smaller, which does not require much work. It has a ratio of 100:5, meaning for every 100 calories of fat you ingest, you burn approximately 5 calories in the digestive process.
- *Complex carbohydrate* takes more effort to digest because of the glucose molecules. It has a ratio of 100:10, meaning for every 100 calories you ingest, you burn about 10 during digestion.
- *Protein* requires about 25 percent more energy to digest because it is made up

Glycemic Index

Most of us are familiar with the glycemic index by now. The glycemic index was designed as a quick and convenient way to find out how fast your blood glucose levels rise after you eat various carbohydrate-containing foods.

Many of us have been told to eat foods that are lower on the glycemic index. What you probably have not have been told is that the glycemic index only applies when the food is consumed by itself. In other words, if you eat a fruit, let's say blueberries, alone, you will get a boost in insulin production (10). However, if you eat the blueberries with some cottage cheese, your insulin production won't increase nearly as much because of the protein in the cottage cheese. So, if you are going to eat fruit, eat it with some protein. Starchy carbs also cause an insulin spike when consumed alone. This is why it's so important to eat complementary meals as described earlier in this chapter.

Additionally, most vegetables, especially green ones, don't do much to elevate your insulin levels. So, go nuts with the green veggies!

of 20 different amino acids—nine of which are essential amino acids supplied through food. It has a ratio of 100:25, meaning for every 100 calories you eat, you burn approximately 25 calories to digest it.[16]

Based on TEF, if most of your meals are complementary, it is easy to see how you end up consuming fewer calories and burning more. Plus, there's no unrealistic dieting and no need for additional calorie counting!

As stated previously, fat loss does come down to calories in versus calories out (i.e. the first law of thermodynamics). And, since one pound of fat has about 3,500 calories, you need a 500 calorie per day deficit in order to lose one pound of fat.[11]

Now, there are two ways to create a caloric deficit. You can either eat less calories or you can eat the same amount of calories and increase your activity level to burn more calories. This is yet another reason why cardio works faster than weight training in these short term studies comparing cardio training to weight training for fat loss fat loss, because cardio burns more calories during the workout than strength training. However, instead of spending the extra time doing cardio to burn (let's say) 300 calories, you can simply cut 300 calories out of your diet each day and end up with the same result without having to bother with all the potential side effects and boredom issues involved with cardio, which I covered in the previous chapter. This is yet another reason why cardio training isn't emphasized in the strength training for fat loss system, as in most cases, you eliminate the need for it (from a fat loss perspective) when you simply eat less calories to create a deficit.

As I stated earlier in the chapter, I don't recommend counting calories right off the bat when you begin integrating in the complementary eating strategy into your normal lifestyle because simply by using this strategy you're eating less calories and burning more. However, if you reach a point where you're using the complementary eating strategy and you're not losing roughly one pound of fat per week, then I say it's time to begin counting your calories to ensure that you're in a caloric deficit needed to lose fat.

It's worth mentioning that just as a caloric deficit is needed to lose fat, a caloric surplus is needed to build muscle. So it stands to reason that one can't build muscle while losing fat. However, keep in mind that stored fat is stored energy, so those stored fat calories are available for the body to use as fuel for the muscle-building process. No! Your body can't turn fat into muscle or vice versa. Fat is fat and muscle is muscle. But, if you're overweight, it can use your stored energy (i.e., stored fat is the caloric surplus) to fuel the muscle-building process when that fuel isn't coming from additional food intake. This is still consistent with the first law of thermodynamics.

However, if you're already fairly lean, a large caloric deficit will generally make you lose some muscle even with strength training and adequate protein.[12,13] So, the goal, for everyone, especially when you're not overweight but just looking to lose that extra bit of fat, is to make sure your diet delivers plenty of protein and that you're doing regular strength training as I've directed you in this book. When you do that you'll limit muscle loss to a very small amount, if any.

THE LOWDOWN ON SUPPLEMENTS

One thing even fitness professionals often have a distorted view of is supplements. Put simply, supplements should be taken *in addition to* something; they are not the thing itself. That said, once you get situated with complementary eating habits and a comprehensive training program, there are a few scientifically proven safe and effective supplements we recommend because they boost your workout performance, which will help to accelerate your fat loss.

Protein

A quality protein powder can serve as the protein part of meal, a snack, or a pre- or postworkout shake. We recommend either a 100 percent whey protein isolate powder or a combination of casein and whey, because research has shown them to be the most superior forms of protein. If for some reason you aren't interested in whey protein, then other supplements such as soy and egg have been shown to be beneficial as well.

To go into all of the specifics about protein is beyond the scope of this book. But, I will tell you that there are lots of myths and misconceptions about protein regarding how much is too much, potential side effects, and so on. I cover the science on protein in *The Protein Report*, which you can download for free at www.freeproteinreport.net.

Creatine

Creatine monohydrate is one of the most researched supplements on the market. It's also one of the most misunderstood—the scientific evidence doesn't line up with many of the common claims we often hear about its side effects or potential dangers.

The science has clearly shown that creatine monohydrate is 100 percent safe for both men and women, and even for kids, and it's effective at boosting your workout performance giving you better results from your workout efforts. Plus, creatine works fast and is affordable. If you'd like more information, I've written a fully comprehensive resource called *The Creatine Report*, which you can get for free at www.freecreatinereport.com.

Caffeine

If you're a coffee drinker like me, you'll love to hear that research has shown

- 400 milligrams or less increase muscle strength and endurance, blunt pain, and burn more fat (14);
- caffeine does help to mobilize fat;
- caffeine does increase your heart rate, but it's a nonissue if you're healthy and free of blood pressure and heart troubles;
- caffeine does *not* dehydrate you; and
- 100 milligrams per day before training will help if you aren't already a regular caffeine user. The more you use caf-

feine, the higher the dosage must be to have an effect.

Here's how I recommend you put these supplements to good use by including them as part of your preworkout nutrition to ensure you get the most out of each and every workout. Around 30 to 60 minutes before training, consume the following:

- 100 to 400 milligrams of caffeine (sources include coffee or supplementation)
- 20 grams of a fast-digesting protein such as whey
- 20 to 40 grams of a slow-digesting carbohydrate such as berries (optional)
- 5 grams of creatine monohydrate

Sure there are a multitude of supplements on the market, but many, like fad diets, are based on good marketing and little-to-no science. So, I caution to stick with the supplements that are highly researched and proven effective—like the ones I listed above. And, do your homework and look into the research on any other supplements before you even think about spending your hard-earned money.

Before wrapping up this chapter, it's important to note that although the title of this book is *Strength Training for Fat Loss*, all of the exercise protocols and programs provided are also great for improving your work capacity (i.e., conditioning). There is usually little to no difference between fat-loss exercises and metabolic conditioning exercises; both are intense in nature and demand a total-body effort for extended periods of time, which is what you get from the workouts provided in this book. The only thing that separates a conditioning program from a fat-loss program is the diet. You most certainly can improve your work capacity without going on any special calorie-restrictive diet. But in order to lose body fat, some diet adjustments need to be made and adhered to (i.e., the 85–15 rule), such as the nutrition advice provided in this chapter.

Splurge Meals

We can't talk about eating for fat loss and not discuss splurge meals. We all have high-fat, high-calorie foods that we love to eat. And, if you want to keep your sanity and you want your (healthy) eating to be manageable, you absolutely must eat those not-so-healthy foods you love every once in a while. My advice is to follow the 85–15 rule. This means that if 85 percent of the time you eat in the way I've described in this chapter, then 15 percent of time you can eat whatever you want. In real world terms, that's about 1 in every 7 meals. And, if you're eating 4 meals per day, that one of your meals every two days. That's how moderation works and that's how you do a no-diet diet!

If you're actively training for a physique show or a sporting competition, then you may need to be stricter than 85–15 for the short time you're in prep phase. But for the most part, life is too short to always be stressed and unhappy because you can't eat the foods that you enjoy.

Finally, as far as follow-through goes, that's on you. No one is perfect and neither are the typical situations life throws at us through work, travel, and family responsibilities. I don't expect every meal you eat to be perfect, and neither should you! Just try to use the simple eating strategies in this chapter to do as best you can, do better than you've done before, and to empower yourself to see through the confusion created by infomercials, conflicting information, fad diets, and confusing industry jargon. It's no wonder even health professionals are confused about what to eat when there are 500-page nutrition books on the shelves that rarely provide more practical eating knowledge than I just did here in a single chapter.

Circuits

Circuit training is a classic metabolic strength training concept that involves multiple exercises, using various training equipment from free-weights to machines to body weight, performed back to back with little rest. Circuit training also forms the foundation of the workout programs featured in this book. This chapter discusses a style that we call *big circuits*.

BIG CIRCUIT TRAINING

Big circuits are sequences that involve three, four, or five bigger compound exercises (i.e., exercises that use a large amount of muscle, as opposed to isolation exercises) with heavier loads. The circuits alternate upper-body exercises with lower-body exercises to ensure that each muscle group can maximally recover, which ensures your ability to maintain maximal workout intensity and optimal control on each exercise and each circuit round. This is crucial because the key to maximizing metabolic cost in these big circuits is working at a consistently high intensity. By the time you get back to training the same muscle group on the following circuit round, it's been several minutes, leaving those muscles plenty of time to fully recover and get ready to exert maximal intensity with every set.

In addition to sequencing upper-body exercises with lower-body exercises in an alternating fashion, unilateral (single-sided) exercises are also used in this circuit training method in the following forms:

- *Left–right circuit:* As the name indicates, this circuit splits the body from left to right. It incorporates unilateral exercises, and it involves performing all reps of a given exercise on the left side of your body before switching sides and performing all reps on right side.

- *Unilateral circuit:* This circuit also incorporates unilateral exercises. However, unlike the left–right circuit, every exercise in the circuit is performed only on one side of the body. Then, all the reps are performed on the other side of the body. A rest break can be taken in the transition between sides.

There are two unique benefits of unilateral strength exercises beyond simply adding muscle and accelerating metabolism. First, you experience increased activation of the core muscles. Any time you hold a heavy load on one side of the body and not the other, it lights up the core muscles to offset the unbalanced load. This means unilateral circuits are both metabolic and core conditioning all rolled into one comprehensive protocol. Second, you can eliminate strength imbalances. Most people have one side that is stronger than the other. Unilateral exercises allow you to focus on one side at a time, which can help you bring up your weak side and build a more balanced body.

The big circuits are structured as follows.

Big Three Circuit

The Big Three circuit is a great place to start if you are a beginner because it involves the fewest exercises of the big circuits. This way you do not overwork yourself while also allowing yourself room to increase your workload—first by adding weight to the exercises within the Big Three circuit and then by adding more exercises using circuits such as the Big Four or Big Five. The Big Three consists of these three stations:

1. Upper-body pulling exercise
2. Lower-body leg or hip exercise
3. Upper-body pushing exercise

Big Four Circuit

The Big Four circuit is the same concept as the previous circuit but with an added lower-body exercise as the fourth station. The Big Four is a great place to start for anyone at an intermediate fitness level (i.e., you are already exercising, but this type of metabolic strength training is new to you) because it allows scalability. In other words, you not only have room to gradually increase the reps for loads used within the Big Four circuit, but you also have room to progress by adding another exercise by moving on to the Big Five circuit. The Big Four circuit consists of these four stations:

1. Upper-body pulling exercise
2. Lower-body leg exercise
3. Upper-body pushing exercise
4. Lower-body hip exercise

Big Five Circuit

The final progression to this circuit concept is the Big Five. In the Big Five, we have added a fifth station that integrates a core exercise. The Big Five circuit is the most demanding of the big circuits because it involves the most exercises, therefore requiring the most total work volume to complete each circuit round. If you are an advanced exerciser—someone who has been doing regular exercise in a similar fashion to this—you can go right to using Big Five circuits. Otherwise, as stated previously, the Big Five circuit is a sequence that you can gradually work up to after you have built your fitness level using the Big Four circuit. The Big Five consists of these five stations:

1. Upper-body pulling exercise
2. Lower-body leg exercise
3. Upper-body pushing exercise
4. Lower-body hip exercise
5. Abdominal/core exercise

Even advanced exercisers and athletes can benefit from incorporating the Big Three or Big Four circuit into their workout plan (see chapter 9). If your workout involves performing metabolic combinations or complexes that require a high amount of work volume, it makes sense to reduce the volume in your circuits by performing the Big Three circuit in order to minimize the risk of overtraining. And if you increase the work volume of your circuit training (i.e., progress from the Big Four to the Big Five), then you are advised to reduce your volume in another strength training complex or combination protocol.

CIRCUITS

Following are free-weight and machine exercises for upper-body pushing, upper-body pulling, lower-body legs and hips, and abdominal muscles that can be incorporated into the circuit training styles discussed previously. Aside from some of the abdominal exercises, body-weight exercises are excluded here because they're covered in the chapter on body-weight training (chapter 7). Additionally, a few isolation exercises are included in this chapter. Also note that many of these exercises are used in the programs in chapter 9, Fat-Loss Workouts.

You can perform the exercises within a given circuit workout either for a specific time frame or for repetitions, as follows:

- 25 to 40 seconds per exercise
- 6 to 12 reps per exercise

You will perform 3 to 5 total rounds per circuit. As stated before, the type of circuit that you use (Big Three, Big Four, or Big Five) is determined by two factors: your fitness level and the work demand of the other exercise protocols of your workout. It's recommended that beginners start with the Big Three and gradually progress to the Big Four and Big Five as their fitness improves. And, to prevent overtraining, if you add volume to your workout via combinations or complexes, you should reduce your work volume in the circuit aspect of that workout.

Each exercise within a given circuit is performed with as little rest as needed between exercises. To ensure continued progression in each circuit workout, you can increase the weight used in the exercises, increase the work time at each station (i.e., exercise), or reduce the rest time between circuits.

Upper-Body Pushing Exercises

Following are a variety of upper-body pushing exercises. These involve taking something that is close to you and moving it farther away from you in a horizontal, diagonal, or vertical direction.

DUMBBELL BENCH PRESS

Lie on a weight bench with your feet flat on the floor, pressing them firmly into the ground to keep you stable. Hold a pair of dumbbells in each hand above your shoulders with your arms straight (see figure *a*). Slowly lower the dumbbells outside your body until your elbows are at a 90-degree angle (see figure *b*). Press the dumbbells back up toward the sky above your shoulders. You may also perform this exercise on an incline bench that is angled approximately 45 degrees.

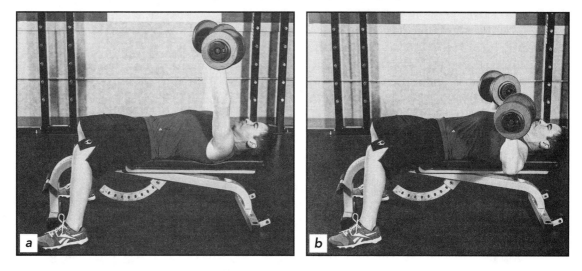

INCLINE DUMBBELL BENCH PRESS

Lie on a weight bench that's angled approximately 45 degrees with your feet flat on the floor, pressing them firmly into the ground to keep you stable. Hold a pair of dumbbells above your head outside your shoulders (see figure *a*). Slowly lower the dumbbells outside your body until your elbows are at a 90-degree angle (see figure *b*). Reverse the motion and press the dumbbells back upward.

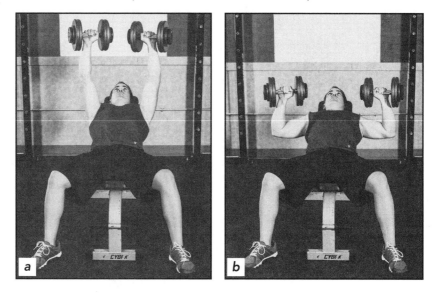

BARBELL BENCH PRESS

Lie on a weight bench with your feet flat on the floor, pressing them firmly into the ground to keep you stable. Unrack an Olympic-style barbell using a grip that places your hands outside your shoulders (see figure a). Slowly lower the bar to your chest, keeping your elbows at a 45-degree angle relative to your torso (see figure b). Press the bar up to the sky above your chest.

As with dumbbells, you can also perform an incline bench press from a weight-bench that's angled at roughly 45-degrees.

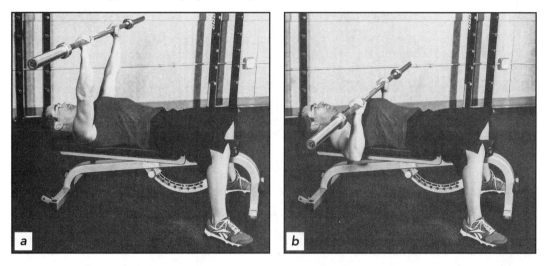

ONE-ARM OVERHEAD DUMBBELL PRESS

Stand tall with your feet roughly shoulder-width apart while holding a dumbbell at shoulder level (see figure a). Press the dumbbell toward the sky, keeping your torso as stable as possible (see figure b). Slowly lower the dumbbell back to your shoulder.

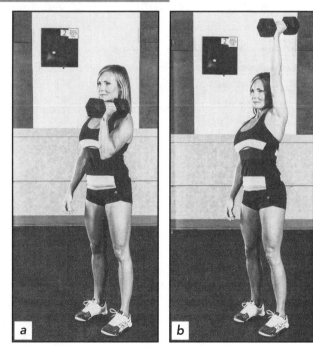

ONE-ARM OVERHEAD DUMBBELL PUSH PRESS

Stand tall with your feet roughly shoulder-width apart while holding a dumbbell at shoulder level (see figure *a*). Slightly bend your knees (see figure *b*) and then quickly reverse the motion, exploding into the dumbbell and driving it overhead using both your arm and legs in a coordinated fashion, pressing the dumbbell toward the sky and keeping your torso as stable as possible (see figure *c*). Slowly lower the dumbbell back to your shoulder.

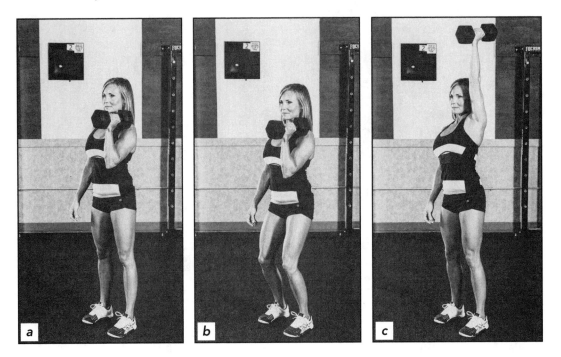

DUMBBELL UPPERCUT

Stand tall with your feet roughly shoulder-width apart while holding a dumbbell in front of each shoulder (see figure *a*). Press one dumbbell into the air as you rotate to the opposite side (see figure *b*). Reverse the motion and press while rotating to the other side. To better allow your hips to rotate in this exercise, raise your heel off the ground as you turn.

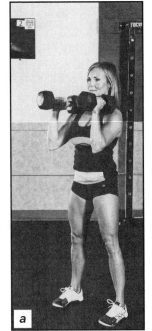
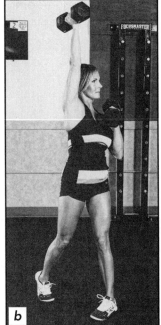

ONE-ARM DUMBBELL UPPERCUT

Stand tall with your feet roughly shoulder-width apart while holding a dumbbell in front of one shoulder (see figure *a*). Press the dumbbell into the air as you rotate to the side opposite the dumbbell (see figure *b*). To better allow your hips to rotate in this exercise, raise your heel off the ground as you turn.

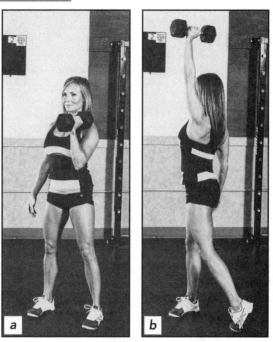

ANGLED BARBELL PRESS

Stand either with your feet parallel to one another and shoulder-width apart or with one leg in front of the other, splitting your stance. Place one end of a barbell in a corner or inside a Sorinex Landmine device (www.sorinex.com) and hold onto the other end of the barbell (see figure *a*). Press it up and away from you without allowing your shoulders or hips to rotate (see figure *b*). Slowly reverse the motion and lower the barbell back to your shoulder.

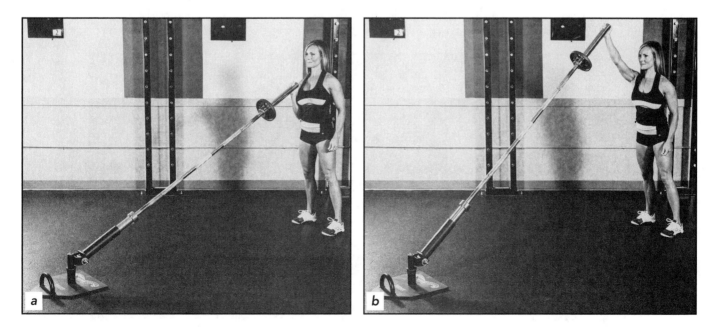

ONE-ARM CABLE PRESS

You'll need an adjustable cable column to perform this exercise. Stand facing away from the cable column holding a handle that's roughly at shoulder height. With the cable handle in your right hand, split your stance with your right leg behind your left leg (see figure a). Press the cable straight out in front of you (see figure b). Slowly reverse the motion and bring the handle back into your body without allowing your shoulders or hips to rotate.

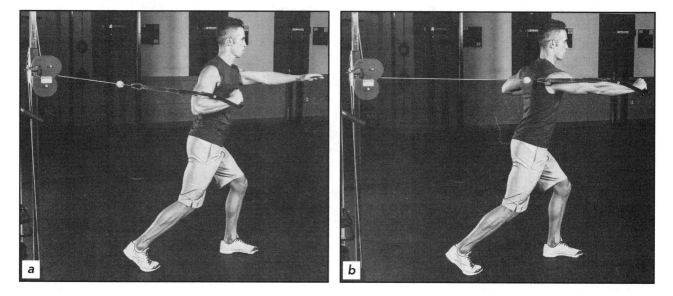

CORE BAR CABLE PRESS

You'll need an adjustable cable column and a core bar to perform this exercise. Stand facing away from the cable column holding the core bar at chest height with your hands wider than shoulder-width apart. With the cable attached to the right side of the core bar, split your stance with your right leg behind your left leg (see figure a). Press the bar straight out in front of you (see figure b). Slowly reverse the motion and bring the bar back into your body without allowing your shoulders or hips to rotate.

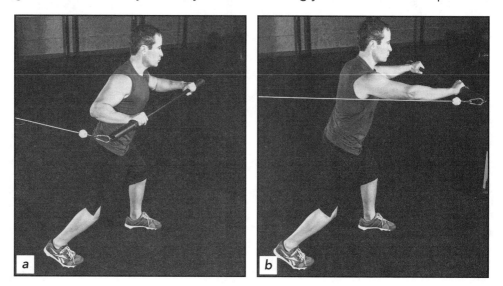

TRICEPS DUMBBELL SKULL CRUSHER

Lie supine on a weight bench holding a dumbbell in each hand with your arms out-stretched above your shoulders toward the sky (see figure a). Bend your elbows, lowering the dumbbells toward your forehead while keeping your palms facing one another (see figure b). Do not allow the dumbbells to hit you in the head. Once your elbows reach a 90-degree angle, reverse the motion and extend your elbows until they're almost straight again to complete 1 rep.

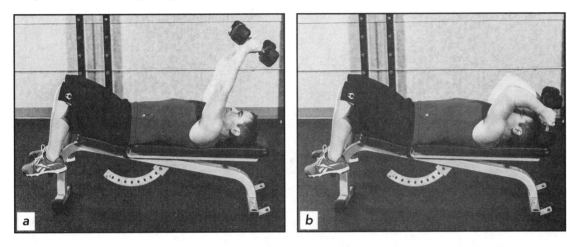

CABLE TRICEPS ROPE EXTENSION

You'll need an adjustable cable column to perform this exercise. Stand in front of the cable column with a rope attached above your eye level. Hold each side of the rope in each hand with your arms by your sides in your elbows bent above 90 degrees (see figure a). With your knees slightly bent, straighten your elbows toward the sides of your body until your arms are straight (see figure b). Be sure not to allow your shoulders to round forward as you press the rope downward on each repetition.

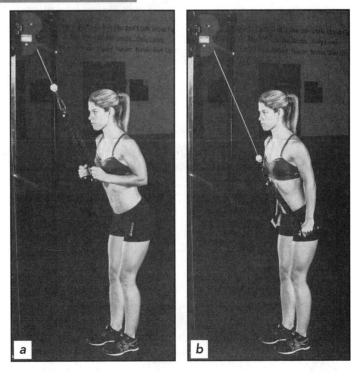

Upper-Body Pulling Exercises

Upper-body pulling exercises are the opposite of the upper-body pushing exercises described previously. These exercises require you to take something that is away from you and pull it closer to you in a vertical, diagonal, or horizontal direction.

CHIN-UP OR PULL-UP

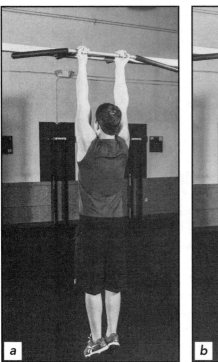
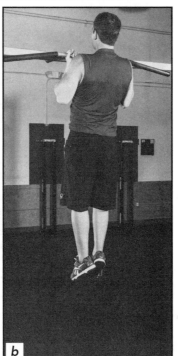

Hang from a straight bar using an underhand grip (see figure a). The underhand grip is usually the strongest grip style for most people. Bring yourself up to the bar (see figure b). Slowly lower yourself under control.

To add variety, you can perform pull-ups by using an overhand grip or varying the widths of the grip you use. You can perform pull-ups either on a straight bar or on a bar that has a slight curve. Another great option is a neutral grip, where your palms are facing one another. Neutral-grip pull-ups require a bar that allows for this grip option. Additionally, some people who experience shoulder discomfort when performing chin-ups or pull-ups find a neutral grip to be more comfortable. And shoulder issues or not, many people simply find the neutral grip to be a stronger option. Experiment with various grips and avoid any that you find uncomfortable.

MACHINE LAT PULL-DOWN

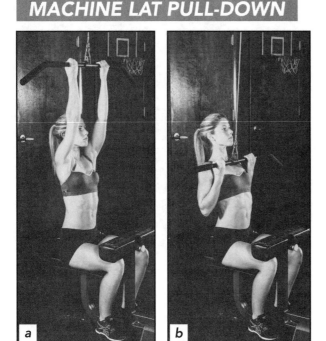

Position yourself immediately behind a traditional lat pull-down bar and hold it with an underhand grip (see figure a). Pull the bar down to the top of your chest while keeping your back straight and elbows following a straight line (see figure b). Slowly reverse the motion under control.

You can also use a wide underhand grip to add difficulty to this exercise. To make the exercise easier, you can use a neutral grip by exchanging the straight bar for a handle that allows your palms to face one another roughly shoulder-width apart. Many people who have minor shoulder issues find the neutral grip to be more comfortable.

T-BAR ROW

Place one end of a barbell in a corner or inside a Sorinex Landmine device and straddle the other end of the barbell. Place a handle that is designed to attach to a seated row or lat pull-down apparatus underneath the barbell below the weight plates. Grab onto each handle with one hand on each side of the barbell (see figure a). Keeping your back straight and your torso stable, row the barbell into your chest and abdomen far as possible (see figure b). Slowly lower the bar until your arms are straight without letting the barbell rest on the ground until the set is over.

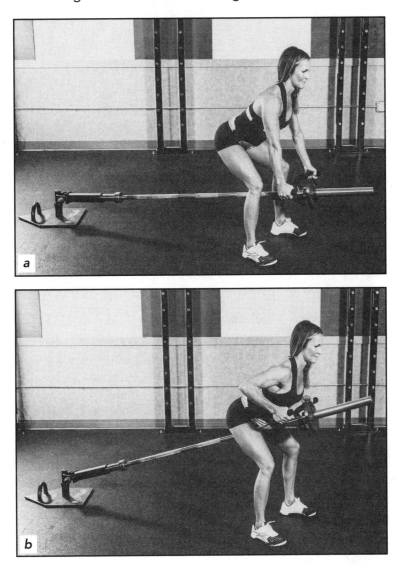

BARBELL BENT-OVER ROW

Stand with your feet roughly hip-width apart. Hold the barbell using an underhand grip, keeping your hands just outside shoulder-width apart. Bend over at your hips, keeping your back straight so that your torso is parallel to the floor and your knees are bent 15 to 20 degrees (see figure *a*). Row the bar into the middle of your torso between your chest and your belly button (see figure *b*). Slowly lower the bar to complete 1 rep. You can also perform bent-over rows by using an overhand grip, which many people find to be a less-strong gripping option.

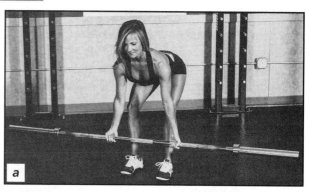

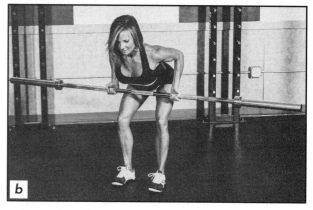

WIDE-GRIP BENT-OVER ROW

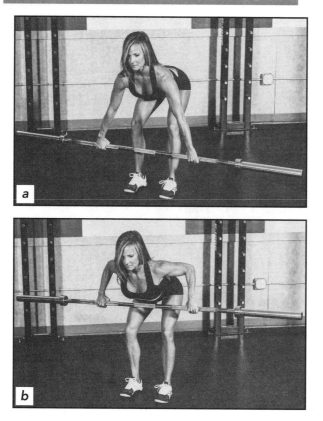

Stand with your feet shoulder-width apart and hold a barbell with your hands roughly 12 inches outside each hip. Bend over at your hips, keeping your back straight so that your torso is parallel to the floor and keeping your knees bent 15 to 20 degrees (see figure *a*). Row the bar into the middle of your torso between your chest and your belly button (see figure *b*). Slowly lower the bar back down without allowing it to contact the floor until the set is completed.

ONE-ARM FREE-STANDING DUMBBELL ROW

Assume a split stance with your right leg in front of your left leg and both knees slightly bent. With your left hand, hold the dumbbell in a neutral position so your palm is facing the opposite side of your body and let your other arm hang at your side. Hinge at your hips, keeping your back straight so that your torso becomes parallel with the floor (see figure a). Perform a row by pulling the dumbbell toward your body without rotating the shoulders or hips while pulling your scapula toward your spine in a controlled manner as your arm moves (see figure b). Be sure to maintain a stable spinal position, keeping your back straight throughout the exercise. Slowly lower the dumbbell without letting it touch the floor. Complete all reps on one side before switching sides.

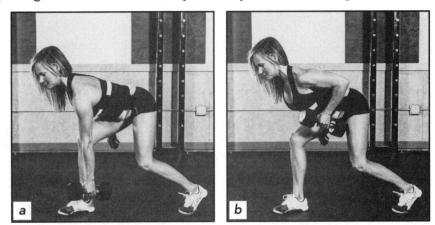

ONE-ARM DUMBBELL BENCH ROW

You will need a traditional gym weight bench to perform this exercise. Stand facing the weight bench with your right hand on top of the weight bench and a dumbbell in your left hand (see figure a). Your feet are hip-width apart, with knees slightly bent and a straight back that is roughly parallel to the floor. Perform the row by pulling the dumbbell toward your body so that your left elbow ends up at roughly a 90-degree angle while you simultaneously drive your left shoulder blade toward your spine (see figure b). Slowly lower the dumbbell toward the floor until your arm straightens without allowing the dumbbell to touch the floor.

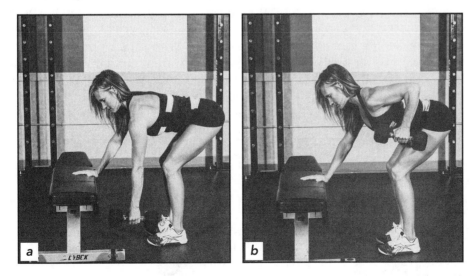

ONE-ARM CABLE ROW

You'll need an adjustable cable column to perform this exercise. Stand tall with your spine straight and in a split stance with your knees slightly bent while facing a cable column that's adjusted to roughly shoulder height. With your left hand, grab the handle in a neutral grip (i.e., palm facing the opposite side of your body) and split your stance so your left leg is behind your right leg (see figure *a*). Perform a row by pulling the cable toward your body, driving your shoulder blade back so that it's retracted at the end range of the row (see figure *b*). Maintain a stable spine without allowing your shoulders and hips to rotate during the exercise. Slowly reverse the motion by allowing your scapula to protract while your arm straightens.

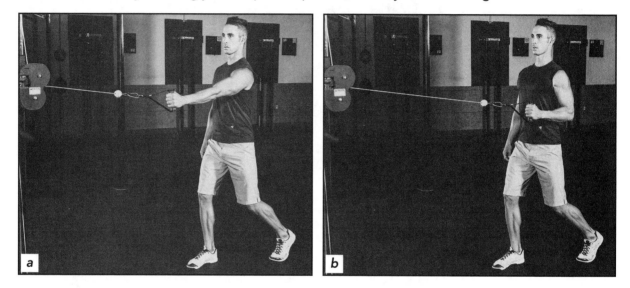

ONE-ARM CABLE MOTORCYCLE ROW

This exercise is performed using an adjustable cable column. Stand in front of the cable column with your feet roughly shoulder-width apart in a split stance with your right leg in front and the cable roughly the same height as your chest. With your left hand, grab the handle in a neutral grip (i.e., palm facing the opposite side of your body) and hinge at your hips with your knees slightly bent so that your torso is parallel with the floor and the cable (see figure *a*). Pull the cable toward your body as you would in a lat pull-down, keeping your working arm in line with the cable (see figure *b*). Perform all the reps on one side before switching to the other side.

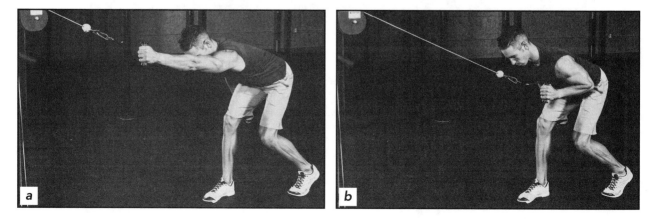

ONE-ARM COMPOUND CABLE ROW

You'll need an adjustable cable column to perform this exercise. Stand facing the cable column with your feet roughly shoulder-width apart in a split stance with your right leg in front and knees slightly bent. With your left hand, hold the handle with a neutral grip (i.e., palm facing the opposite side of your body) (see figure a). Hinge at your hips, reaching your left arm above you toward the origin of the cable (see figure b). Reverse this motion while simultaneously performing a row (see figure c). You'll finish the row at the same time you return to standing upright. Slowly reverse the motion, hinging at your hips and reaching out using good rhythm and timing. Perform all the reps on one side before switching to the other side.

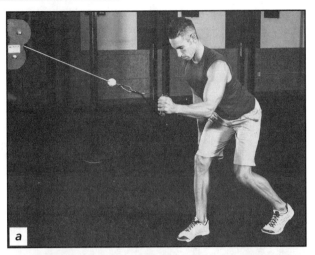

a

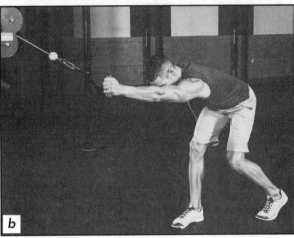

b

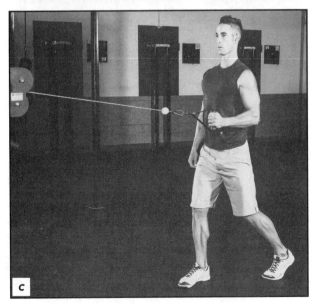

c

CORE BAR CABLE ROW

You'll need an adjustable cable column and a core bar to perform this exercise. Stand facing the cable column holding the core bar at about shoulder height with your hands wider than shoulder-width apart. With the cable attached to the left side of the core bar, split your stance with your left leg behind your right leg (see figure *a*). Pull the core bar into your body with your left arm while keeping your right elbow slightly bent (see figure *b*). Slowly reverse the motion by allowing your left arm to straighten without allowing your shoulders or hips to rotate.

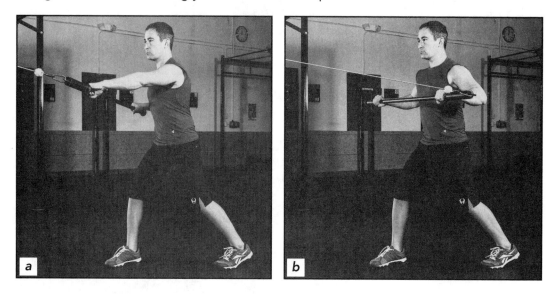

SEATED ROW

This exercise requires a specially designed seated row apparatus that is available in most gyms. Sit on the seat with your feet hip-width apart against the platform with your knees slightly bent and your back straight. Hold the handles using a neutral grip (or a wide grip using a lat pull-down bar) (see figure *a*). Pull the handles into your body (see figure *b*). Slowly reverse the movement. Be sure that you do not overarch your lower back as you row.

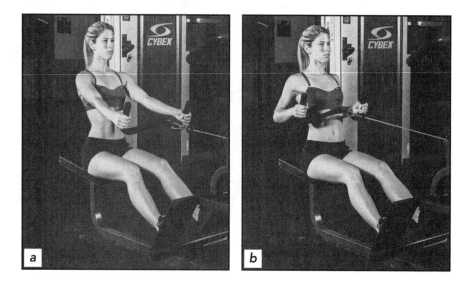

MACHINE REAR DELTOID FLY

This exercise requires a specially designed machine that is available in most gyms. The machine allows you to pull its handles horizontally to the outside of your body. Sit tall with your chest in front of the pad and hold the handles with a neutral, over-hand, or underhand grip depending on the gripping options the machine allows (see figure a for an example using the neutral grip). Find a comfortable foot place-ment that best allows you to perform the exercise with proper technique. Keeping your elbows slightly bent, open your arms out to the sides of your body (see figure b). Slowly reverse the movement. Be sure to keep a stable spine and minimize any overarching in your lower back when performing this exercise.

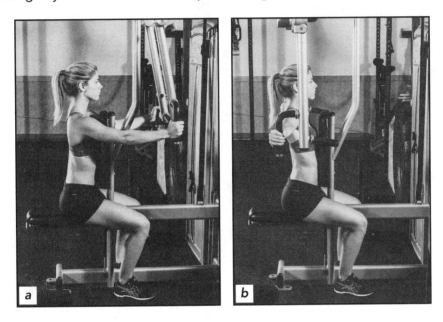

DUMBBELL BICEPS CURL

Stand tall with your feet hip-width apart, holding a dumbbell in each hand by your hips (see figure a). Curl the dumbbells up toward your shoulders by bending at your elbows without allowing your elbows to move forward (see figure b). Once your hands are up in front of your shoulders, reverse the motion by slowly lowering the dumbbells to your sides. You can also perform dumbbell biceps curls by alternating your arms.

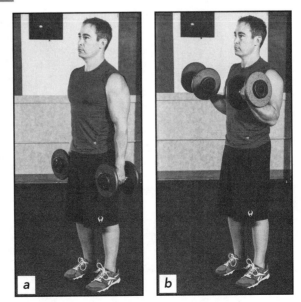

CABLE BICEPS ROPE CURL

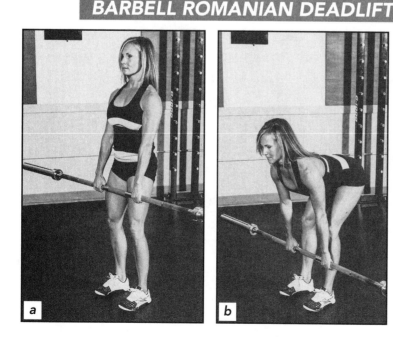

You'll need an adjustable cable column to perform this exercise. Stand in front of the cable column with a rope attached below your knees. Hold each side of the rope in each hand with your arms by your sides in your elbows slightly bent (see figure a). With your knees slightly bent, bring your hands toward your shoulders (see figure b). Be sure not to allow your elbows to move forward as you curl the rope in on each repetition.

Hip-Oriented Lower-Body Exercises

Because the muscles that make up the lower body are often all involved when performing compound lower-body exercises, it becomes difficult in many cases to associate any compound lower-body exercise with specific lower-body muscles. That said, some lower-body compound exercises involve more movement at your hip joint than at your knee joint. These are what we classify as hip-oriented lower-body exercises. Here is a wide-variety of hip-oriented lower-body exercises that are used in this system of strength training for fat-loss.

BARBELL ROMANIAN DEADLIFT

Stand tall with your feet hip-width apart, holding a barbell in front of your thighs with your arms straight (see figure a). Keeping your back straight, hinge at your hips and bend forward toward the floor, keeping your knees bent at a 15- to 20-degree angle (see figure b). As you hinge forward, drive your hips backward and do not allow your back to round out. Once your torso is roughly parallel to the floor or the weight plates lightly tap the floor, drive your hips forward toward the barbell, reversing the motion to stand tall again and complete 1 rep.

ONE-LEG BARBELL ROMANIAN DEADLIFT

This is the single-leg version of the Romanian deadlift and is performed using the same mechanics as the double-leg Romanian deadlift. Stand on one leg while holding a barbell in front of the weight-bearing thigh with your arms straight (see figure a). Keeping your back straight, hinge at your hip and bend forward toward the floor, keeping the weight-bearing knee bent at a 15- to

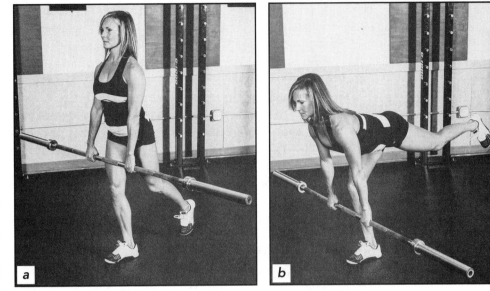

20-degree angle (see figure b). As you hinge, allow your non-weight-bearing leg to elevate upward so it remains in a straight line with your torso. Be sure to keep your lower back from rounding out. Once your torso and non-weight-bearing leg are roughly parallel to the floor or the weight plates lightly tap the floor, drive your hips forward toward the barbell, reversing the motion to stand tall again and complete 1 rep.

You can also perform this exercise with a pair of dumbbells (or one dumbbell) using the same technique; however, performing it with a barbell requires more stability than dumbbells because it's more difficult to counteract the shift of a long barbell to one side than it is to manage the dumbbells. So if you have difficulty with balance, try using dumbbells.

ONE-LEG ONE-ARM DUMBBELL ROMANIAN DEADLIFT

Stand on one leg and hold a dumbbell in the opposite hand (see figure a). Keeping your back and arm straight, hinge at your hip and bend forward toward the floor, keeping your weight-bearing knee bent at roughly a 15- to 20-degree angle (see figure b). As you hinge, allow your non-weight-bearing leg to elevate upward so it remains in a straight line with your torso, and do not allow your lower back to round out. At the bottom position (when your torso is roughly parallel to the ground), be sure to keep your hips flat and do not allow them to rotate. Once your torso and non-weight-bearing leg are roughly parallel to the floor, reverse the motion by driving your hips forward to stand tall again, completing 1 rep.

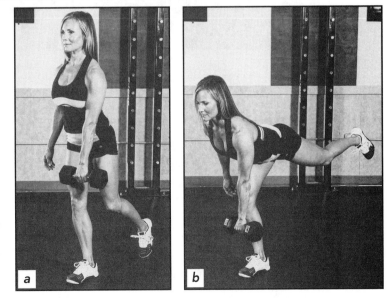

ONE-LEG 45-DEGREE CABLE ROMANIAN DEADLIFT

This exercise is performed exactly like the one-leg Romanian deadlift with a dumbbell, except it uses a cable column on the low setting to change the vector of resistance to a 45-degree angle. Stand on one leg, holding the cable handle in your opposite hand (see figure *a*). Keeping your back and your arm straight, hinge at your hip and bend forward toward the floor, keeping your weight-bearing knee bent at a 15- to 20-degree angle (see figure *b*). As you hinge forward, allow your non-weight-bearing leg to elevate upward so it remains in a straight line with your torso. Be sure to keep your lower back from rounding out. At the bottom position (just before your torso is parallel to the ground), keep your hips flat and do not allow them to rotate. Once your torso and non-weight-bearing leg are roughly at a 45-degree angle to the floor, reverse the motion by driving your hips forward toward the cable to stand tall again and complete 1 rep.

Note that the range of motion is shorter when using the cable because the force you are working against is at a higher point than when using the dumbbell. The dumbbell is pulling you toward the floor, whereas the cable is pulling you toward it or at a 45-degree angle.

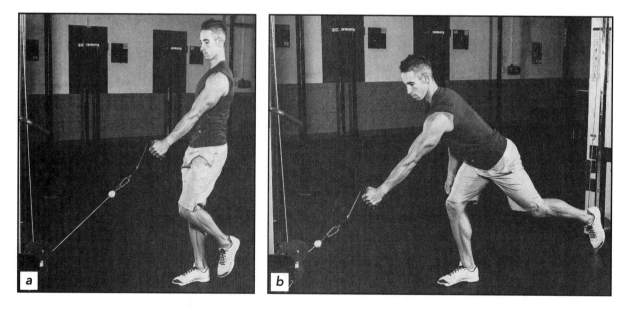

BARBELL GOOD MORNING

Stand tall with your feet hip-width apart and place a barbell across your shoulders behind your head (see figure a). Keeping your back straight, hinge at your hips and bend forward toward the floor, keeping your knees bent at roughly a 15- to 20-degree angle (see figure b). As you hinge forward, drive your hips backward and do not allow your back to round out. Once your torso is roughly parallel to the floor, drive your hips forward toward the barbell, reversing the motion to stand tall again and complete 1 rep.

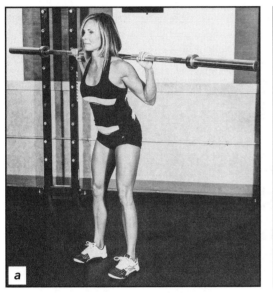
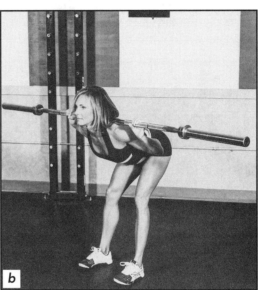

KETTLEBELL SWING

The kettlebell swing is performed using the same mechanics as the Romanian deadlift. The only difference is this movement is performed at a greater speed. With your feet shoulder-width apart, hold a kettlebell with both hands. Keeping your back and arms straight, drive the kettlebell between your legs as if hiking a football and hinge forward at your hips, keeping your knees bent at roughly a 15- to 20-degree angle (see figure a). Once your forearms come into contact with your thighs, explosively reverse the motion by simultaneously driving your hips forward (see figure b) and swinging the kettlebell upward to eye level to complete 1 rep.

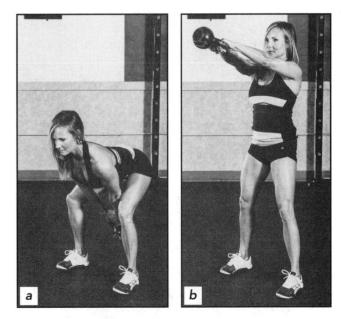

BARBELL BENCH HIP THRUST

Sit on the floor with your back against a weight bench and a barbell over the top of your hips. Bend your knees 90 degrees, keeping your legs roughly hip-width apart (see figure *a*). Drive your hips toward the sky as far as possible without overarching at your lower back (see figure *b*). At the top position your hips should be roughly the same height as your shoulders so your body forms a tabletop-like position. Slowly lower your hips to the floor and repeat. Make sure that the bench your shoulders are resting on is supported by something stable before you perform this exercise. Also, wrap the barbell with a thick towel or use a thick bar pad to make this exercise more comfortable on your hips. If you don't have a bench, you can also perform this exercise while lying on the floor.

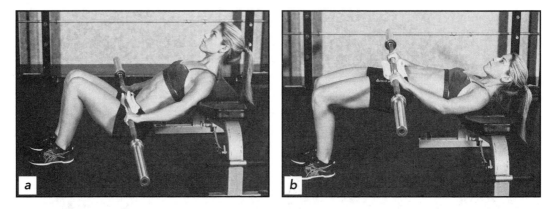

ONE-LEG HIP THRUST

Sit on the floor with your shoulders elevated on a weight bench or chair, rest your head and shoulders on the bench and open your arms to the sides with palms facing up. Position with your legs out so that your knees are bent at about 90 degrees and your feet are directly below your knees. Keeping your right knee bent 90 degrees, lift it above your hip (see figure *a*). Lift your hips so that your body makes a straight line from knees to nose (see figure *b*). Keeping your right leg lifted, lower your hips toward the floor to complete 1 rep. You can make this move more difficult by adding weight—try holding a weighted bar across your hips.

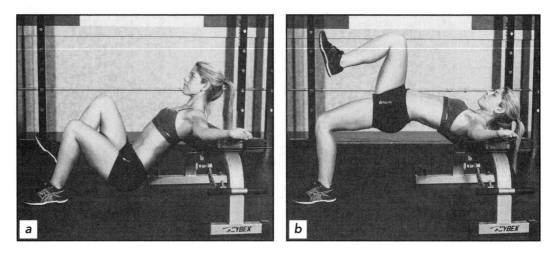

HORIZONTAL HIP EXTENSION

To perform this exercise, you will need a specially designed apparatus known as a back extension machine. Rest your thighs against the pad so that the pad is positioned below your hip bones and cross your arms in front of your chest (see figure a). With your feet hip-width apart, hinge at your hips, keeping your back straight (see figure b). Reverse the motion by extending at your hips without overarching your lower back to pull yourself up so that your body forms a straight line from shoulders to hips to ankles. You can also perform a unilateral version of this exercise by removing one leg and placing it over the ankle pad instead of underneath.

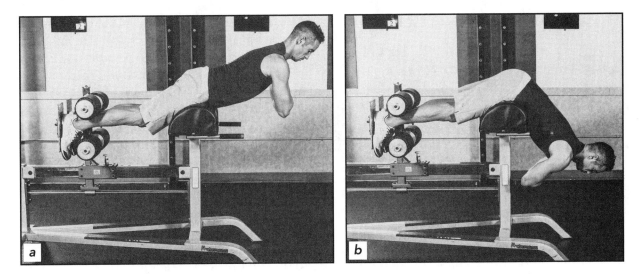

REVERSE HORIZONTAL HIP EXTENSION

To perform this exercise, you will need a specially designed apparatus known as a back extension machine. Facing the back of the machine, lie across the top, grabbing onto the back of the machine so your legs hang down without allowing your lower back to round (see figure a). With your feet hip-width apart, hinge at your hips lifting your legs up so that your body forms a straight line (see figure b). As you raise your legs also allow your feet to move farther apart while keeping your legs straight.

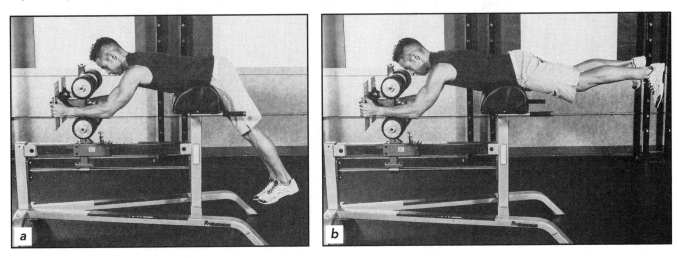

DUMBBELL ANTERIOR-LEANING LUNGE

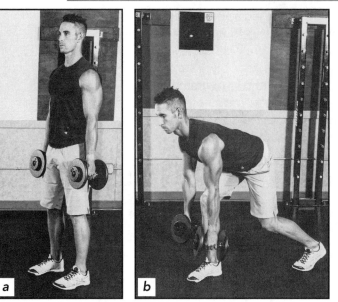

Stand tall holding dumbbells by your sides with your feet hip-width apart (see figure a). Step forward with one leg, keeping your front knee bent 15 to 20 degrees and your back knee straight or slightly bent. As your front foot hits the ground, lean forward by hinging at your hips and allowing your rear heel to come off the ground (see figure b). Your torso should be no more than parallel to the floor and your back should be straight. Reverse the motion by stepping backward so your feet are together again and you return to an upright position. Then perform the same motion stepping forward with the other leg. Do not let the dumbbells touch the floor at any point during this exercise.

DUMBBELL BULGARIAN SPLIT SQUAT

Stand tall holding dumbbells by your sides. Place your left foot on top of a bench or chair behind you in a split-squat stance (see figure a). Lower your body toward the floor without allowing your back knee to rest on the floor (see figure b). As you lower your body, keep your back straight and lean your torso slightly forward at roughly a 45-degree angle. Drive your heel into the ground to raise your body to the starting position to complete 1 rep. Perform all reps on one side before switching to the other leg.

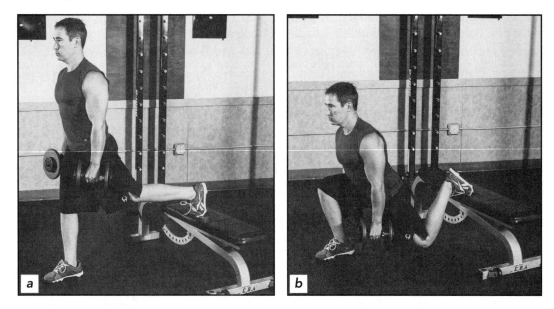

LYING HAMSTRING CURL

To perform this exercise, you'll need to use the machine that's commonly known as the lying hamstring curl or lying leg curl machine. Assume a lying position with your hip joint on top of the apex of the pads. Adjust the pad you'll be pushing against to a position that's at the bottom of your calves (see figure *a*). Hold onto the handles, and with your legs hip-width apart, pull your heels toward your glutes as far as possible (see figure *b*). Slowly reverse the motion under control.

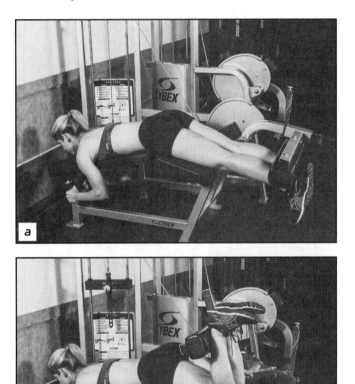

Leg-Oriented Lower-Body Exercises

In order to ensure a well-rounded workout program, we not only want to do lower-body exercises that primarily involve movement at the hip joint, but we also want to include lower-body exercises that emphasize movement at the knee joint, otherwise known as leg-oriented exercises. Following are leg-oriented lower-body exercises that are used within this system of strength training for fat loss.

BARBELL BACK SQUAT

Place a barbell across your shoulders (not on top of your neck) and stand with your feet just wider than shoulder-width apart with your toes turned out 10 to 15 degrees (see figure a). Bend at your knees and hips and lower your body toward the floor as low as you can possibly go (see figure b). Your heels should not to lift off the ground and your lower back should not lose its arch. Also, be sure to keep your knees wide and tracking in the same direction as your toes. Do not allow your knees to drop in toward the midline of your body. Once you've gone as deep as you can control in the squat, reverse the motion and stand up.

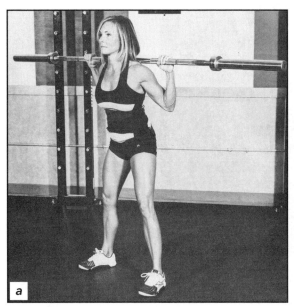

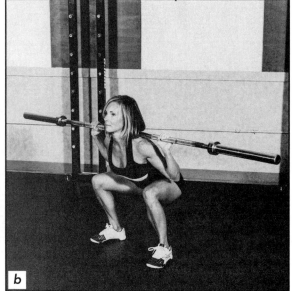

BARBELL FRONT SQUAT

The front squat is performed using the same mechanics as the back squat; the only difference is the bar placement. Rest an Olympic-style barbell on top of your chest and stand with your feet just wider than shoulder-width apart with your toes turned out 10 to 15 degrees (see figure a). Be sure to stay tall and lift your chest to create a rack for the bar instead of trying to hold the bar up using only your arms. Bend at your knees and hips and lower your body toward the floor as low as you can possibly go (see figure b). As you drop into the squat, be sure to keep your elbows lifted high toward the sky. Your heels should not lift off the ground and your lower back should not lose its arch. Also, be sure to keep your knees wide and tracking in the same direction as your toes. Do not allow your knees to drop in toward the midline of your body. Once you've gone as deep as you can control in the squat, reverse the motion and stand up.

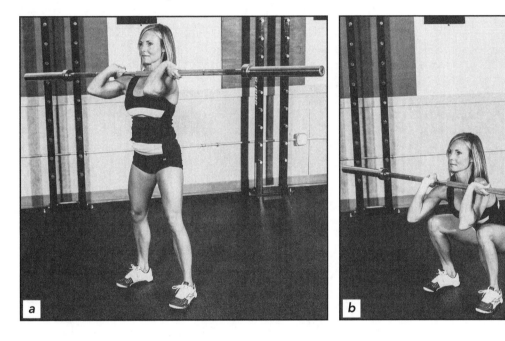

TRAP BAR SQUAT

To perform this exercise, you need a specially designed bar commonly known as a trap bar. Although this bar is a fantastic piece of equipment because it offers a unique squat exercise variation, it is not commonly found at most gyms. That said, I am including it here to encourage you to use it just in case you do have access to a trap bar.

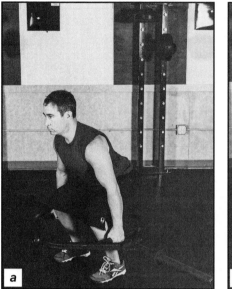

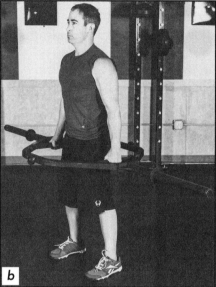

Stand inside the bar with your feet at roughly shoulder-width apart in a squatting position with your hands holding onto the handles (see figure a). Be sure to keep your feet flat, your knees in line with your toes, and a strong lordodic arch in your lower back. Stand up tall so that your hands end up directly outside of your hips (see figure b). Slowly lower back into the squat until the weight plates you have loaded on the bar touch the floor or until you can no longer maintain the optimal arch in your lower back.

GOBLET SQUAT

Stand tall with your feet shoulder-width apart with your toes turned out slightly, about 10 degrees (see figure a). Hold a dumbbell vertically on your chest with both

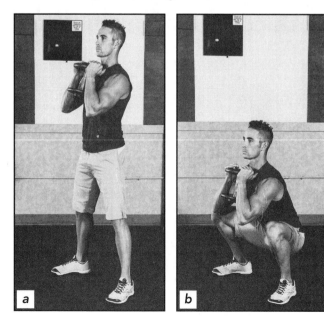

hands. Clamp the dumbbell by pressing your elbows together. Perform a squat by bending your knees and sitting back at your hips (see figure b). Go as low as you can possibly go without allowing your lower back to round out. Be sure that as you squat you do not allow your heels to come off the ground or your knees to come together toward the midline of your body. Your knees should track in the same direction as your toes.

DUMBBELL WALKING LUNGE

With your feet hip-width apart, hold a pair of dumbbells, one in each hand (see figure a). Take a large step forward and drop your body so your back knee lightly touches the floor (see figure b). Stand back up tall while simultaneously bringing your rear leg forward to meet your front leg and step forward with the opposite leg, the one that was behind you on the last rep (see figure c). A slight forward torso lean with a straight spine instead of an upright torso at the bottom of each lunge is okay because it's a bit easier on your knees (the slight forward lean helps recruit your glutes). Repeat as you move down the room.

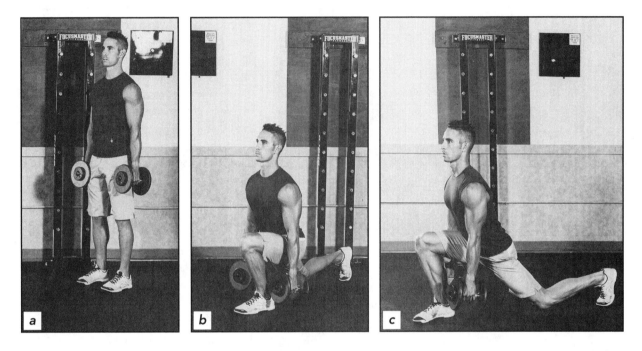

DUMBBELL REVERSE LUNGE

The mechanics of the reverse lunge are the same as in the walking lunge, except you don't move across the room and you step backward instead of forward. With your feet hip-width apart, hold a pair of dumbbells, one in each hand (see figure a). Step backward with your left foot and drop your body so your knee lightly touches the floor (see figure b). Reverse the movement by coming out of the lunge and bringing your left foot forward so that you are back to your starting position. Perform the same movement on the opposite leg.

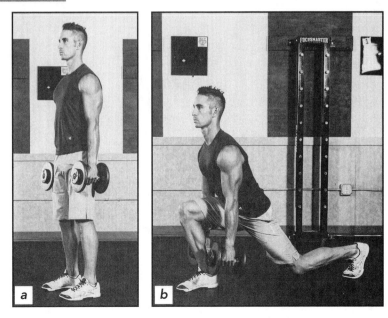

SLIDER SPLIT SQUAT

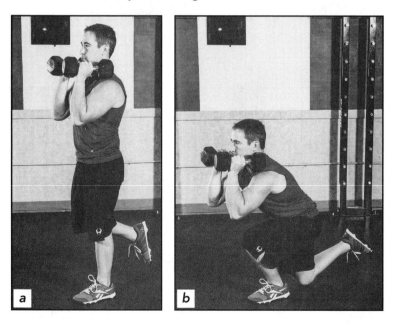

The movement and mechanics of the slider split squat are the same as in the reverse lunge, except in this case you perform all reps on one leg because your other foot (on the nonworking side) is on a slider, paper plate, or anything else that allows you to slide your foot across the floor. Holding a pair of dumbbells, one in each hand, place your left foot on top of a slider or a paper plate, keeping your heel up (see figure a). Drive your left leg backward and lower your body into a reverse lunge position (see figure b). Reverse the motion by coming out of the lunge and pulling your back foot to meet your other foot. Perform all reps on one side before switching and repeating on the other side.

KNEE-TAP SQUAT

Stand with your right knee bent and slightly behind your left leg, and your hands outstretched in front of you as a counterbalance (see figure a for an example using a dumbbell). Slowly lower yourself toward the floor and lightly tap your back knee on the object (see figure b). Reverse the motion and stand up again. It's okay if you can't squat deep enough to allow your back knee to touch the object that's behind you. Squat as low as you possibly can without allowing your back (non-weight-bearing) foot to touch the floor. You can also remove the 4- to 6-inch object to increase the range of motion and touch your knee to the floor on each rep.

You can also perform this exercise holding a dumbbell at each shoulder (see figures a and b). Also, using a 4- to 6-inch box can make the exercise easier. Perform all reps on the same leg before switching sides.

DUMBBELL BENCH STEP-UP

Stand with your feet hip-width apart facing a weight bench, holding a dumbbell in each hand by your hips. Place your left foot on top of the bench (see figure a), and step up by extending your left knee (see figure b). Once at the top of the bench, allow your right foot to gently come in contact with the bench to help maintain your balance, then reverse the motion by stepping down with your right foot touching the ground first. Then bring your left foot down to the floor and place your right leg on top of the bench to repeat with the other leg. Essentially, you are stepping up and down using the same leg each time, and you are switching the working leg—the leg you are stepping with—on the ground, not when you're on top of the bench.

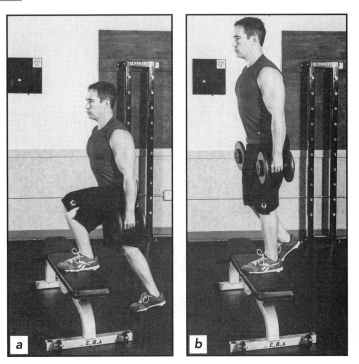

Abdominal Exercises

So far we've covered the movements dictated by your extremities: upper-body pushing and pulling along with lower-body leg and hip exercises. Now it's time to focus on those muscles that make up your center: your abdominal muscles.

Although this section provides exercises that emphasize your abdominal musculature, the exercise applications also involve your shoulders and hips. Also note that exercises such as Romanian deadlifts, front squats, one-arm shoulder presses, and angled presses could also be considered core exercises because your core is not just your abdominal muscles but all of the muscles that make up your torso, and the exercises just listed, as well as several others described previously, require you to use various muscles of your torso in order to maintain your body alignment. For example, squats and deadlifts both require your lower-back musculature to work to resist the weight of the barbell pulling you forward and causing your back to round out, and muscles such as your obliques on the left side of your body must work to control your torso and keep you centered while performing a one-arm overhead press or an angled barbell press on your right side.

In other words, many of the exercises provided thus far stimulate the posterior and lateral torso muscles. What the following exercises do is serve as a nice complement to the previous exercises by focusing on the anterior torso muscles: the abdominal muscles.

DUMBBELL PLANK ROW

In a push-up position with your feet shoulder-width apart, hold a dumbbell in each hand directly under your shoulders (see figure *a*). Row one dumbbell up into your body until it touches your ribs (see figure *b*). Slowly lower the dumbbell to the floor and row the other dumbbell in the same manner. Be sure that your torso remains as stable as possible and you do not allow your hips to rotate at any time.

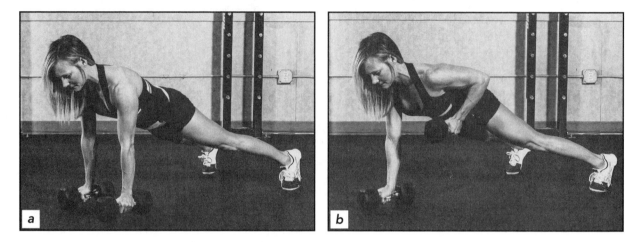

SIDE PLANK TO DUMBBELL LATERAL RAISE

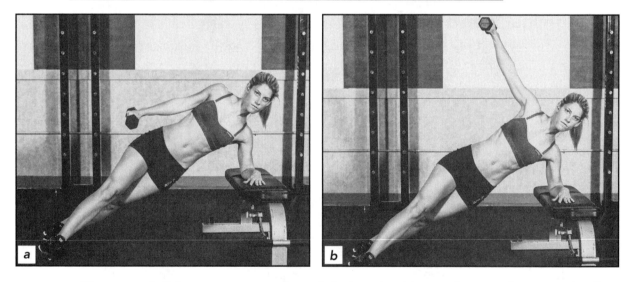

Place your left forearm on top of a weight bench with your feet on the ground split apart one in front of the other (see figure *a*). Keep a straight line with your entire body from your nose to your belly button to the middle of your legs. This is the side elbow plank position. Maintain this position while you perform the side shoulder raise with a dumbbell that you're holding in your right hand. Begin with your right hand in contact with your right hip and raise your arm into the air toward the ceiling, keeping your elbow fairly straight, until your arm ends up over your shoulder (see figure *b*). Slowly lower your hand back to your hip. Repeat all reps on same side before switching sides.

ONE-ARM FARMER'S WALK

With your feet hip-width apart, hold a fairly heavy dumbbell on one side of your body at your hip (or at your shoulder) with your palm facing your body (see figure a). Walk up and down the room, keeping the dumbbell in this position while maintaining a strong upright posture (see figure b). Then switch hands and repeat by holding the dumbbell on the other side.

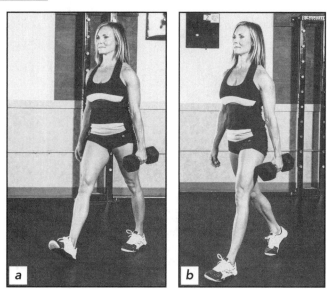

TURKISH GET-UP

Although the Turkish get-up has a single name, it is truly a combination of several exercises that can be done while holding a dumbbell (or kettlebell). If you've never tried the Turkish get-up, get ready for an exercise that's unlike any other.

Lie supine on the floor, holding a dumbbell (or kettlebell) in your left hand. Reach your arm toward the sky directly above your shoulder and bend your left knee (see figure a). Roll to your right elbow, keeping your left arm stable (see figure b). Then extend your right elbow to sit up (see figure c). Raise your hips into the air (see figure d) and slide your right leg underneath your body (see figure e), placing your right knee on the floor while continuing to keep your left arm straight and stable (see figure f). Then raise your torso so that it's perpendicular to the floor (see figure g). Finally, stand up out of the half-kneeling position (see figure h). Then slowly reverse each motion step by step until you're in the starting position in order to complete 1 rep. Repeat on the other side. Note that you can switch hands after each rep or switch sides every two, three, or four reps and so on—whatever you feel is needed to maintain optimal intensity and control when performing the exercise.

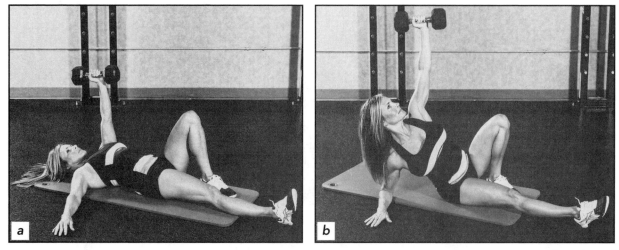

(continued)

(continued)

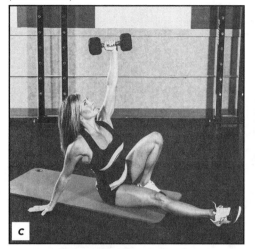

c

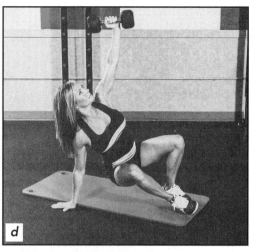

d

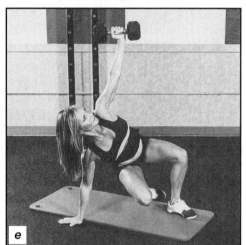

e

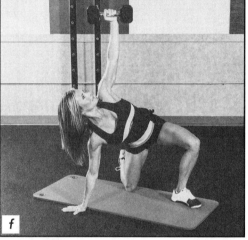

f

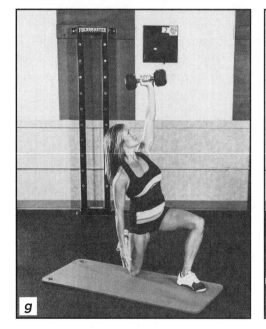

g

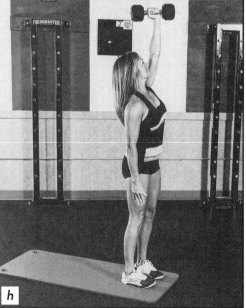

h

ANGLED BARBELL RAINBOW

Place one end of a barbell in a corner or into a Sorinex Landmine device and hold the other end of the barbell with both hands while you stand tall with your feet roughly shoulder-width apart. Move the barbell from side to side in a rainbow-like arc while you rotate your hips and shoulders and maintain a straight spine allowing your torso to face the barbell at all times. (see figures a-c).

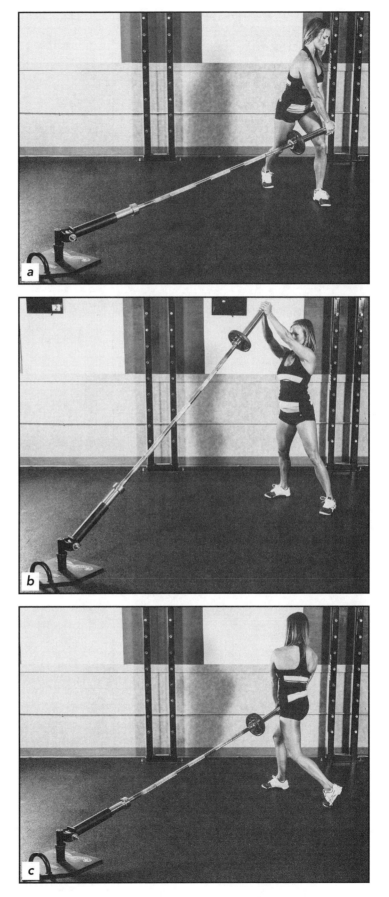

ANGLED BARBELL TIGHT RAINBOW

Place one end of a barbell in a corner or into a Sorinex Landmine device and hold the other end of the barbell with both hands while you stand tall with your feet roughly shoulder-width apart. Move the barbell from side to side in a rainbow-like arc from one shoulder level to another without allowing your any rotation at your torso and maintain a straight spine (see figures a-c). As you move the barbell from side to side, your torso should always remain facing the end of the barbell that is anchored.

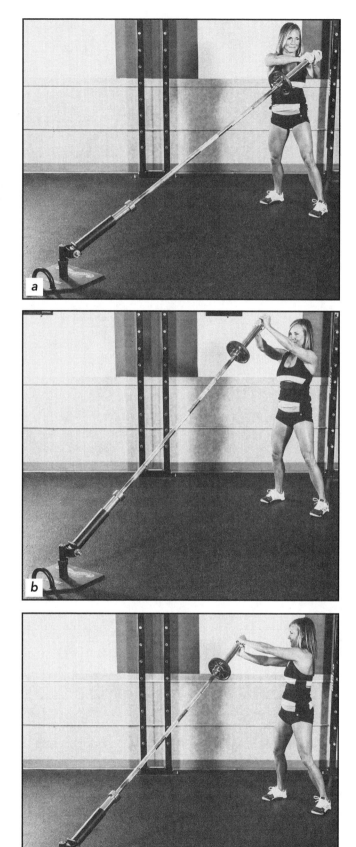

BALL ROLL-OUT

Kneel on the floor with your arms straight and your palms on a 55- to 65-centimeter stability ball with your knees and hands hip-width apart (see figure *a*). Drive the ball away from you by extending your arms overhead as if you were diving into a pool (see figure *b*). Push the ball out as far as you can without allowing your head or lower back to sag toward the floor (see figure *c*). Once you've gone as far as you can or your arms are completely up overhead in a straight line with your torso, reverse the motion and pull the ball back to the starting position where your hands are just above your head. To make this exercise easier, simple begin with your forearms resting on top of the ball, and perform the rest of the exercise as described.

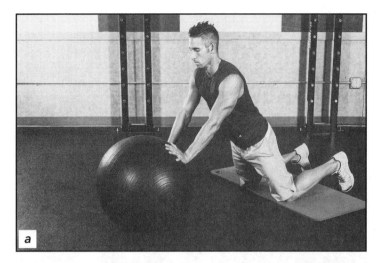

a

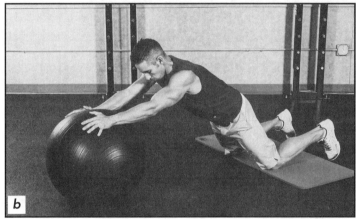

b

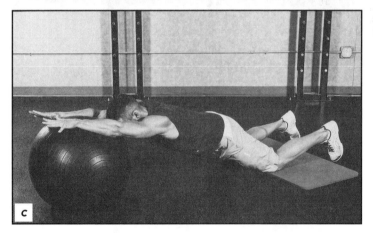

c

STABILITY BALL STIR THE POT

Place both forearms on top of a fitness ball and assume a plank position with your body in a straight line and your feet shoulder-width apart (see figures a and b). Move your arms in small circles (see figures c and d). Alternate between clockwise and counterclockwise circles without allowing your head or hips to sag toward the floor.

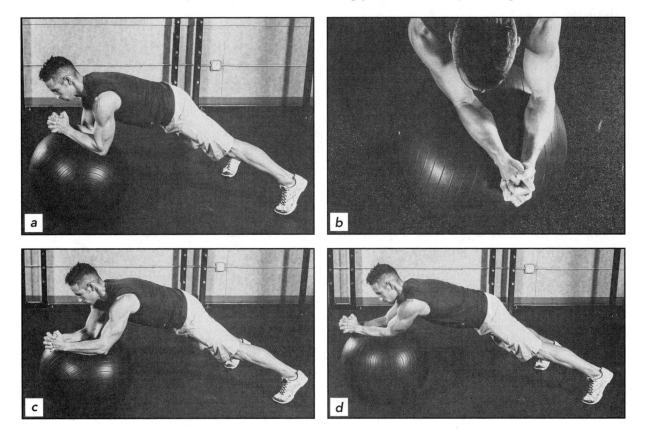

BALL KNEE TUCK

Assume a push-up position with your feet resting on top of a fitness ball that's between 55 and 65 centimeters in size (see figure a). Take your knees in toward your body as far as you possibly can without allowing your shoulders to move away from above your wrists where they started (see figure b). Reverse the motion so your body becomes straight again to complete 1 rep.

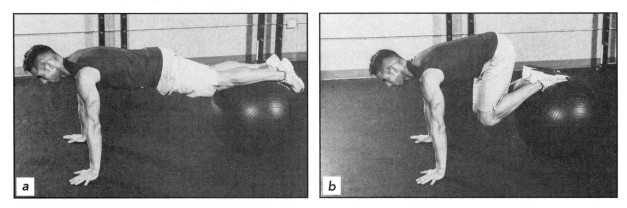

BALL PIKE

Assume a push-up position with your feet resting on top of a fitness ball that's between 55 and 65 centimeters in size (see figure a). Use your abs to raise your hips toward the sky, keeping your legs fairly straight. Raise your hips until just before they reach above your shoulders (see figure b). Slowly lower to the starting position with your body straight.

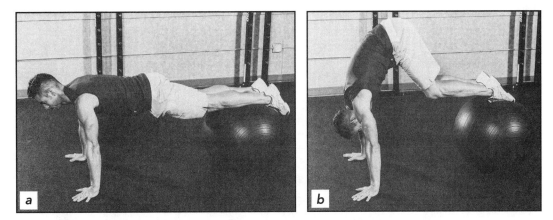

BALL PIKE ROLLBACK

This exercise combines the ball pike in the ball rollout into one comprehensive abdominal exercise. Hold yourself in a push-up position with your feet on a Swiss ball that's between 55 and 65cm in size (to make the exercise easier, move the Swiss ball toward your belly button). With your body in a plank position (see figure a), keep your legs straight and push your hips toward the ceiling while keeping your back flat (see figure b). After straightening your hips and coming back to the start position, push your body backward on the ball until your arms are fully extended in front of you and your legs are fully extended behind you (see figure c). Reverse the motion and repeat.

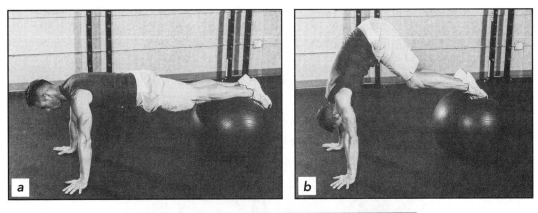

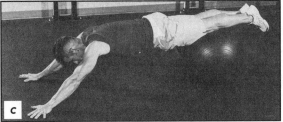

BALL PLATE CRUNCH

Lie down with a fitness ball in the arch of your lower back and hold a weight-plate directly above your chest with your arms outstretched (see figure *a*). Perform a crunch, reaching the weight-plate toward the sky (see figure *b*). Slowly reverse the motion, allowing your abdominal muscles to stretch over the ball. When performing this exercise, be sure that the ball does not roll at any point. Also, do not sit all the way up so that your torso is perpendicular to the floor, because this takes the tension off your abs.

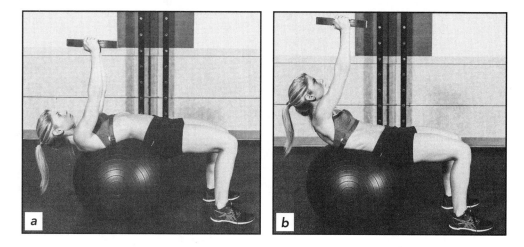

CABLE TIGHT ROTATION

To perform this exercise, you'll use an adjustable cable column. Stand with your feet shoulder-width apart with the handles of the cable on your right side. Grab the handles on your right side with your elbows slightly bent (see figure *a*) and pull them across your body toward the left until both arms are just outside your left shoulder (see figure *b*). Move your arms horizontally in the opposite direction (toward the origin of the cable or band) until they reach just outside your opposite shoulder. The range of motion in this exercise is small, roughly the same as the width of your shoulders. Be sure that you remain tall and do not allow your hips to rotate—they should remain perpendicular to the cable origin throughout.

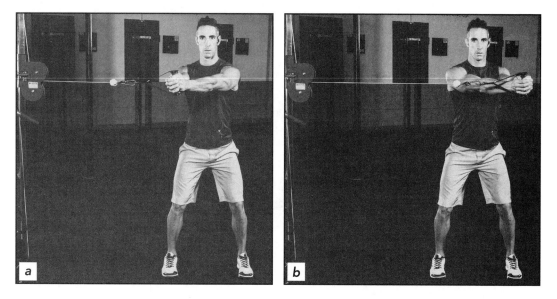

CABLE HIGH CHOP

Stand with your feet slightly wider than shoulder-width apart and perpendicular to a cable column that is on one side, holding the handle with both hands; the handle should be attached to the lowest position. Squat down while simultaneously shifting most of your weight to the leg closest to the column while your arms are at a downward angle reaching toward the origin of the cable (see figure *a*). Stand up while simultaneously shifting your weight toward the other leg as you also drive the cable at a diagonally upward angle across your body (see figure *b*). Finish at the top with your arms above your head on your side. Reverse the motion to the starting position and repeat. Be sure to keep your spine in a neutral position throughout the exercise and to set your hips back at the bottom position.

Your torso should remain fairly perpendicular to the cable column. Do not rotate your torso away from the cable column as you reach the top of the range of motion of the exercise. Doing so greatly reduces the tension on your torso muscles. Perform this exercise both eccentrically and concentrically in a smooth and coordinated fashion. You may also perform this exercise using a resistance band attached at a low position.

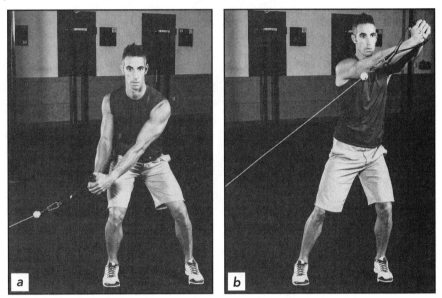

REVERSE CRUNCH

Lie supine on the floor with your knees bent and hips flexed into your belly. With your elbows slightly bent, hold on to a dumbbell or medicine ball that's resting on the floor above your head (see figure *a*). In a smooth controlled fashion perform a reverse crunch by rolling your lower back up off of the floor driving your knees toward your chin (see figure *b*). Slowly reverse this motion allowing your back to lower toward the floor one vertebrae at a time. Be sure to not use momentum and jerk your body in order to perform this exercise. Additionally, hold on to a dumbbell or medicine ball that is heavy enough to not allow you to lift it off of the ground while performing this exercise. Furthermore, your legs should not extend and your head should not lift off of the ground at any point during this exercise.

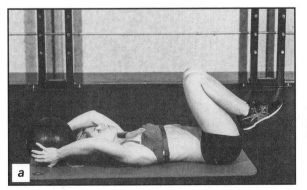
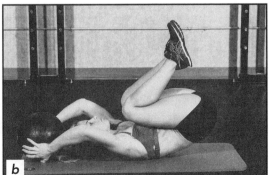

LEG LOWERING

Lie supine on the floor with your knees bent and hips flexed and fists on each side of your head pressing into the floor (see figure *a*). Slowly lower your legs toward the floor keeping your knees bent and pressing your fists into the floor, without allowing your lower back to come off the floor. Once your heels lightly touch the floor, reverse the motion bringing your knees back above your hips. To make this exercise more challenging simply extend your legs out farther as you lower them toward the floor. Put simply, the farther you straighten your legs, the harder the exercise. Just make sure that you never allow your lower back to lose contact with the floor at any point.

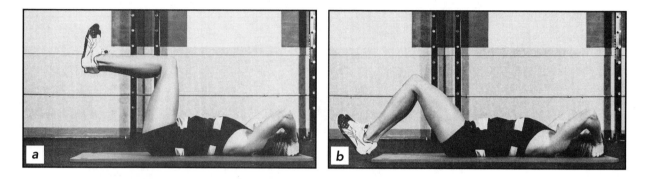

Clearly, circuit training is an extremely versatile and useful metabolic weight training method. As shown in this chapter, you have not only a wide variety of exercises you can use as part of a circuit, but also various ways you can structure your big circuits.

Combinations

As the name implies, strength training combinations involve multiple strength training movements blended together in a seamless fashion to make one exercise. This chapter covers a multitude of strength training combinations involving barbells, dumbbells, cables, and the core bar.

COMBINATION TRAINING

The metabolic strength combinations featured in this chapter have been inspired by Olympic weightlifting concepts where several barbell movements are combined to perform one Olympic lift. Although the concept of combinations has its roots in Olympic lifting, you don't have to be a trained Olympic weightlifter to perform any of the combinations in this chapter. Additionally, although some of the barbell exercises in the combinations feature Olympic-inspired exercises (such as cleans), in this book the intention of these exercises is not to lift maximum weights with maximum power but to simply add more versatility to various combinations in order to make them more interesting, dynamic, and metabolic. This book has simply taken the concept of combinations and run with it, taking the exercises far beyond the barbell by providing combinations using dumbbells and kettlebells in both bilateral and unilateral protocols.

Most people, even personal trainers, don't understand that total-body *workouts* and total-body *exercises* aren't necessarily the same thing. A total-body workout simply means you've hit all your major body parts within a given workout. On the other hand, a total-body *exercise* uses all of your major body parts within 1 repetition. Metabolic strength training combinations are total-body exercises in the purest sense because they force every joint in your body to work together to perform 1 repetition of the combination. Metabolic strength training circuits (covered in the previous chapter) and complexes (covered in the next chapter), on the other hand, involve performing clusters of various exercises, each of which focuses on a different muscle group, one after the other. For this reason, the workout programs in this book combine combinations along with circuits and complexes to make each workout as comprehensive and effective as possible for creating a total-body training effect that gets you leaner, looking better, and moving better.

In addition, each combination involves using the same piece of equipment and the same weight load, which makes it a useful training option when you're at a crowded gym. With metabolic strength training combinations, you grab one piece of equipment and use it to train your entire body.

COMBINATION EXERCISES

Following you will find a variety of metabolic strength training combinations. Some combinations involve more movements to complete 1 repetition than others. The more movements within a given combination, the tougher it is.

Before we get into the combinations, let's first take a look at how exactly you'll use them. Strength training combinations are used in two ways in the training system put forth in this book.

Combination Method 1

The first method is a timed set, which involves performing as many repetitions as possible of a given combination exercise for one 6- to 10-minute time frame. If performing a unilateral (one side at a time) complex, split the time frame in half and work 3 to 5 minutes per side. After finishing the full time frame, rest 3 to 4 minutes before starting a new exercise protocol.

Combination Method 2

The other method of using combinations takes the more traditional approach, which uses a preset number of sets and reps. This method consists of performing 3 to 5 sets (per combination) for 6 to 10 reps. Then you rest 60 to 90 seconds between sets of a given combination. If you're doing a unilateral (one side at a time) combination, perform 6 to 10 reps per side and then rest approximately 30 seconds before switching sides. Once you've done both sides, completing 1 round, rest approximately 90 seconds before starting the next round.

When using combinations, make sure the load is heavy enough to create an appropriate challenge for the number of reps you're using but not so heavy that it prevents you from controlling the weight or from completing the desired reps. Ensure continued progression by increasing the load, increasing the reps, or reducing the rest time.

Barbell Exercises

No matter how much scientific research is generated or how many modern training methods are developed, basic resistance training continues to reign supreme, with the barbell serving as one of the most effective pieces of exercise equipment available today. Following are various metabolic combinations using a barbell.

Bent-Over Row ▪ Romanian Deadlift
Hang Clean ▪ Overhead Push Press

1 BENT-OVER ROW

Stand with your feet roughly hip-width apart. Hold the barbell using an underhand grip, keeping your hands just outside shoulder-width apart. Bend over at your hips, keeping your back straight so that your torso is parallel to the floor and your knees are bent 15 to 20 degrees (see figure a). Row the bar into the middle of your torso between your chest and your belly button (see figure b). Slowly lower the bar without allowing the barbell to touch the ground. You can also perform bent-over rows by using an overhand grip, which many people find to be a less strong gripping option. Note: After finishing your bent-over rows, place the barbell on the floor and switch to an overhand grip to perform the Romanian deadlift and the rest of the exercises in this combination.

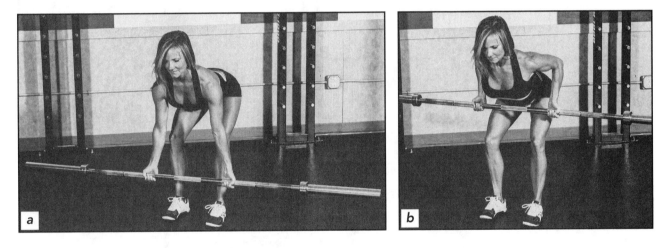

2 ROMANIAN DEADLIFT

Stand tall with your feet hip-width apart, holding a barbell in front of your thighs with your arms straight (see figure c). Keeping your back straight, hinge at your hips and bend forward toward the floor, keeping your knees bent at a 15- to 20-degree angle (see figure d). As you hinge forward, drive your hips backward and do not allow your back to round out. Once your torso is roughly parallel to the floor or the weight plates lightly tap the floor, drive your hips forward toward the barbell, reversing the motion to stand tall again.

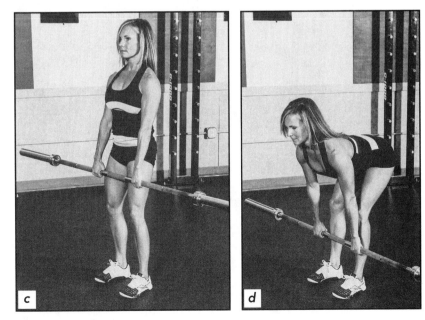

❸ HANG CLEAN

Stand with your feet shoulder-width apart and hold a barbell with your hands just outside shoulder-width apart. Slightly hinge at your hips, keeping the bar against your thighs (see figure *e*), and explode your hips into the bar as you simultaneously pull the bar upward (see figure *f*). Once the bar reaches shoulder level (see figure *g*), quickly flip your elbows underneath the bar to catch it at the top of your chest (see figure *h*).

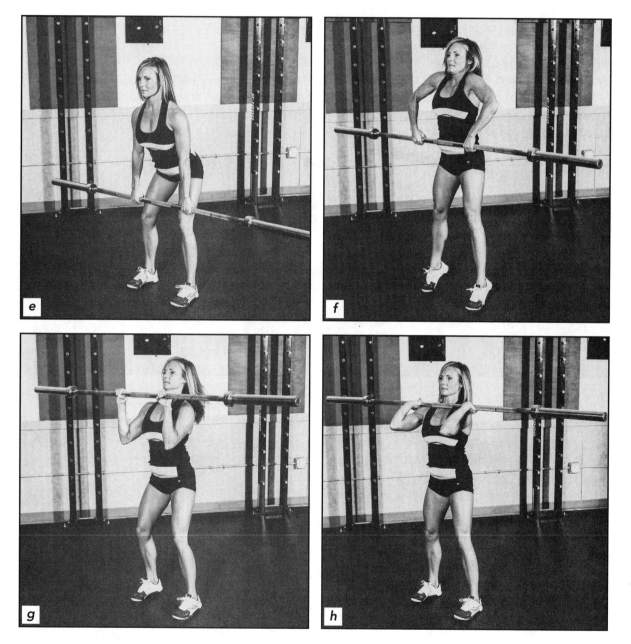

4 OVERHEAD PUSH PRESS

Stand with your feet shoulder-width apart and hold the barbell with your hands just outside shoulder-width apart (see figure *i*). Slightly bend your knees (see figure *j*) and then quickly reverse the motion, exploding into the bar and driving it overhead using both your arms and legs in a coordinated fashion (see figure *k*). Once the bar is completely overhead, slowly reverse the previous motions, replacing the bar on the floor to complete 1 full repetition.

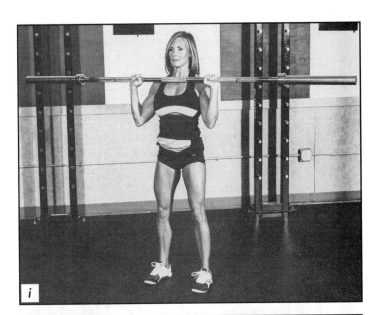

i

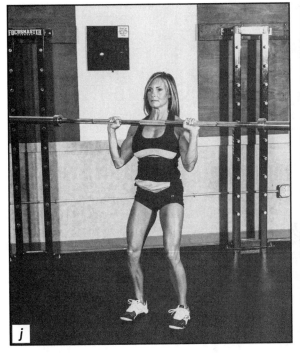

j

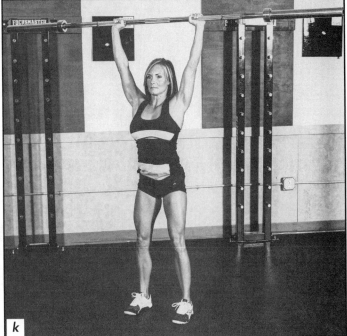

k

Bent-Over Row ■ Romanian Deadlift ■ Jump Shrug ■ Hang Clean ■ Overhead Push Press

1 BENT-OVER ROW

Stand with your feet roughly hip-width apart. Hold the barbell using an underhand grip, keeping your hands just outside shoulder-width apart. Bend over at your hips, keeping your back straight so that your torso is parallel to the floor and your knees are bent 15 to 20 degrees (see figure a). Row the bar into the middle of your torso between your chest and your belly button (see figure b). Slowly lower the bar without allowing the barbell to touch the ground. You can also perform bent-over rows by using an overhand grip, which many people find to be a less strong gripping option.

Note: After finishing your bent-over rows, place the barbell on the floor and switch to an overhand grip to perform the Romanian deadlift and the rest of the exercises in this combination.

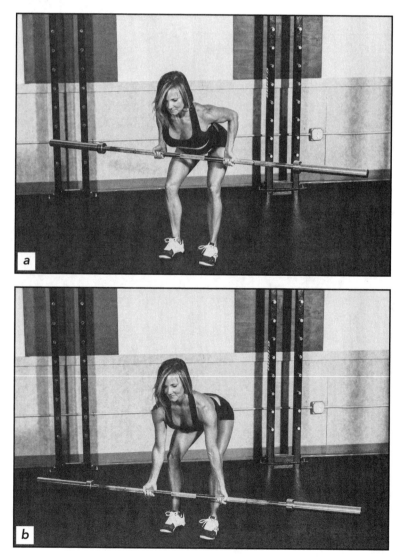

2 ROMANIAN DEADLIFT

Stand tall with your feet hip-width apart, holding a barbell in front of your thighs with your arms straight (see figure c). Keeping your back straight, hinge at your hips and bend forward toward the floor, keeping your knees bent at a 15- to 20-degree angle (see figure d). As you hinge forward, drive your hips backward and do not allow your back to round out. Once your torso is roughly parallel to the floor or the weight plates lightly tap the floor, drive your hips forward toward the barbell, reversing the motion to stand tall again.

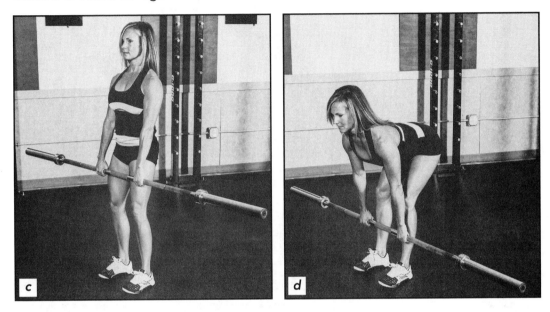

3 JUMP SHRUG

After completing the bent-over row, stand tall (see figure e) and take a small jump into the air as you simultaneously shrug the bar, driving your shoulders toward your ears (see figure f).

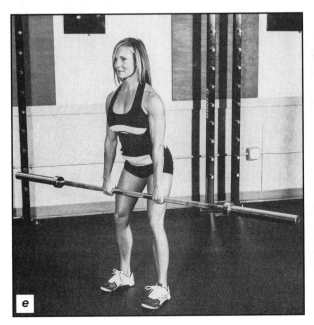
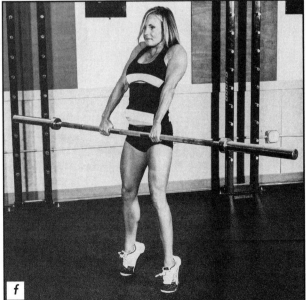

4 HANG CLEAN

Stand with your feet shoulder-width apart and hold a barbell with your hands just outside shoulder-width apart (see figure g). Slightly hinge at your hips, keeping the bar against your thighs, and explode your hips into the bar (see figure h) as you simultaneously pull the bar upward (see figure i). Once the bar reaches shoulder level, quickly flip your elbows underneath the bar to catch it at the top of your chest (see figure j).

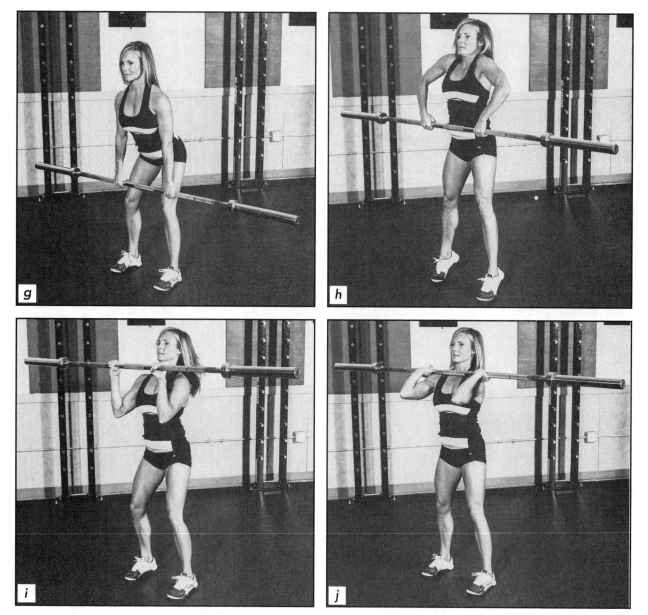

5 OVERHEAD PUSH PRESS

Stand with your feet shoulder-width apart and hold the barbell with your hands just outside shoulder-width apart (see figure *k*). Slightly bend your knees (see figure *l*) and then quickly reverse the motion, exploding into the bar and driving it overhead using both your arms and legs in a coordinated fashion (see figure *m*). Once the bar is completely overhead, slowly reverse the previous motions, replacing the bar on the floor to complete 1 full repetition.

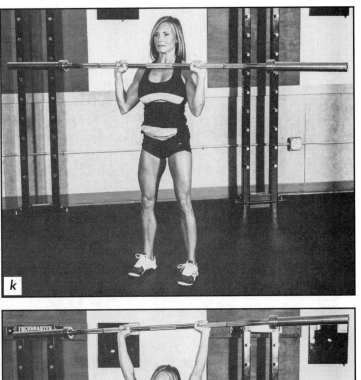

k

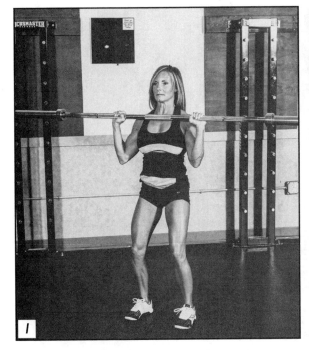

l

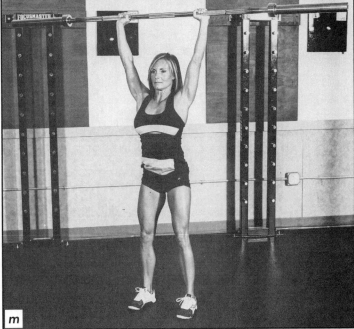

m

Wide-Grip Romanian Deadlift ▪ Wide-Grip Bent-Over Row ▪ High Pull

1 WIDE-GRIP ROMANIAN DEADLIFT

Stand with your feet shoulder-width apart and hold a barbell in front of your thighs with your arms straight and your hands placed on the bar roughly 12 inches outside each hip (see figure *a*). Keeping your back straight, hinge at your hips and bend forward toward the floor, keeping your knees bent at roughly a 15- to 20-degree angle (see figure *b*). As you hinge forward, drive your hips backward and do not allow your back to round out.

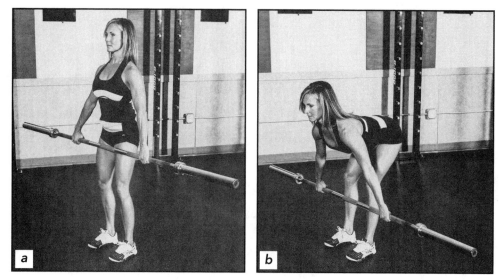

2 WIDE-GRIP BENT-OVER ROW

Stand with your feet shoulder-width apart and hold a barbell with your hands roughly 12 inches outside each hip. Bend over at your hips, keeping your back straight so that your torso is parallel to the floor and keeping your knees bent 15 to 20 degrees (see figure *c*). Row the bar into the middle of your torso between your chest and your belly button (see figure *d*). Slowly lower the bar and then stand tall.

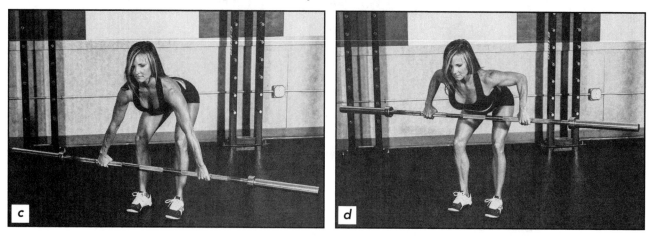

❸ HIGH PULL

Slightly bend your knees and hinge forward at your hips with the barbell resting on your thighs (see figure e). Explode your body upward, pulling the bar toward the sky using your arms and legs simultaneously until your elbows reach shoulder height (see figure f). Then lower the bar back to your thighs in a controlled fashion to reset and begin your next repetition.

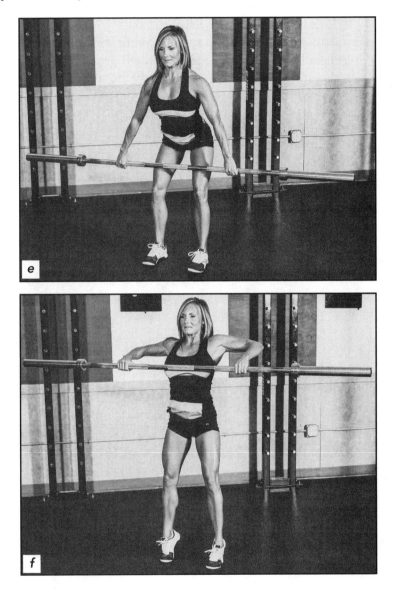

Angled Clean ▪ Angled Rotary Press

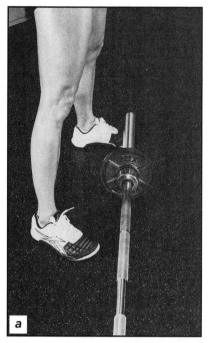

This exercise combination can be performed by placing a barbell in a corner or inserting one end of a barbell into a Sorinex Land-mine device (www.sorinex.com). Following are the exercises for this combination.

1 ANGLED CLEAN

Stand with your feet shoulder-width apart over the weighted end of the barbell (with the weight plates loaded on the end of the barbell) closest to the inside of your left foot (see figure a). Hold the end of the barbell using a mixed grip, taking an overhand grip with your right hand and an underhand grip with your left hand and lower your body into a deadlift position by bending your knees and hinging forward at your hips while keeping your back straight (see figure b). Stand up, lifting the bar off the floor while simultaneously exploding your hips forward into the bar (see figure c) and using your arms to pull the bar to your left shoulder so that the end of the barbell is in front of your chest and your elbows are underneath it (see figure d).

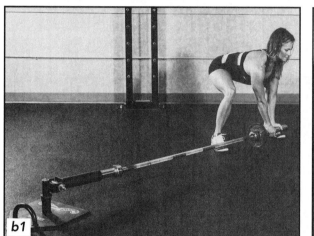

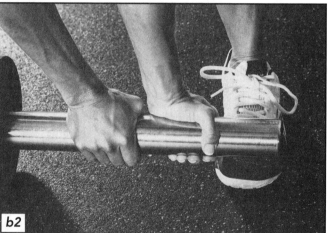

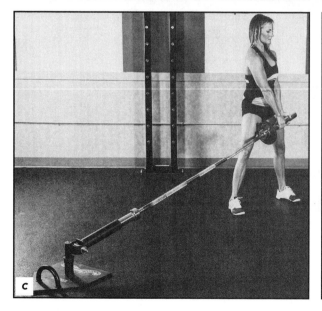

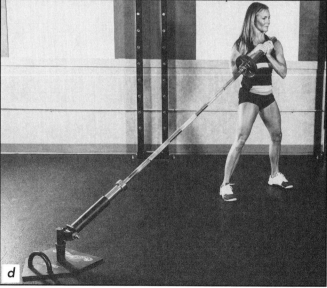

❷ ANGLED ROTARY PRESS

Stand with your feet shoulder-width apart and with the bar at your chest (see figure *e*). Rotate your body (hips and torso) toward the where the barbell is anchored as you push it away from you by extending both arms straight (see figure *f*). Slowly reverse the motions by first lowering the barbell to your chest and then to the floor to complete 1 rep.

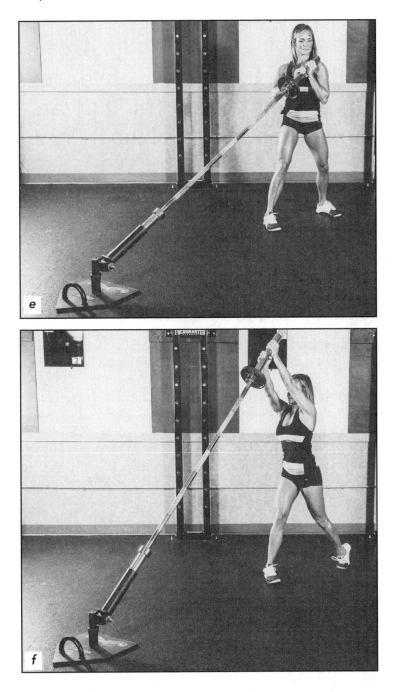

Dumbbell Exercises

There are two unique benefits of using dumbbells. One is that dumbbells allow you to more accurately fit the movement to your arms in the way you are most comfortable instead of having your hands remain in the same place as occurs when using a barbell. The other is that dumbbells allow you to load only one side of your body at a time. When you hold one dumbbell on one side and nothing on the other, you create what is called an *offset load*. When using an offset load, your torso muscles automatically have to kick in in order to maintain your body's alignment.

Freestanding One-Arm Row ▪ Suitcase Squat ▪ One-Arm Assisted Hang Clean ▪ One-Arm Overhead Push Press

This combination is unilateral, meaning that you hold a dumbbell on one side of your body and perform each of the exercises within the combination on that same side. After you've finished performing 1 rep of each of the four exercises in this combination, switch the dumbbell to the opposite hand, position your body properly for the first exercise, and repeat the sequence. You can also perform all reps on the same side first before switching sides. Following are the exercises for this combination.

1 FREESTANDING ONE-ARM ROW

Assume a split-stance position, with one leg in front of the other with both knees slightly bent, and hold a dumbbell in the hand on the back leg side. Hinge at your hips, keeping your back straight so that your torso becomes parallel with the floor (see figure *a*). Perform a row, pulling the dumbbell toward your body without rotating the shoulders or hips, making sure to pull your scapula toward your body in a controlled manner as your arm moves into your body (see figure *b*). Be sure to maintain a stable spinal position, keeping your back straight throughout the exercise. Slowly lower the dumbbell toward the floor without letting it touch the floor.

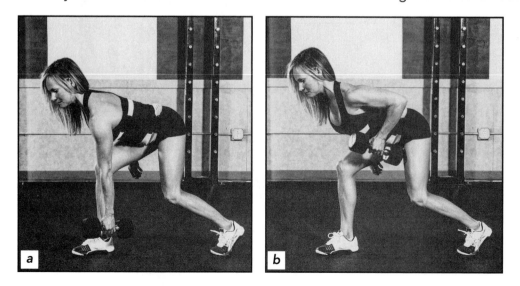

2 SUITCASE SQUAT

With your feet shoulder-width apart, hold a dumbbell in one hand by your hip (see figure c). Bend your knees, sit your hips backward, and lower your body toward the ground while keeping your back from rounding out (see figure d). Once the dumbbell is below the midpoint of your shin, reverse the motion and stand up tall to complete 1 rep.

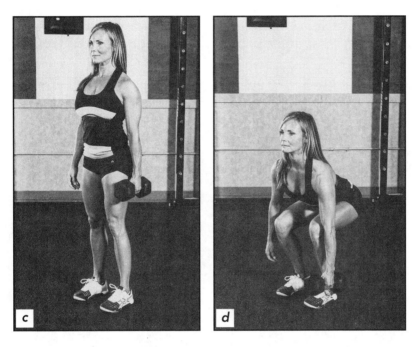

❸ ONE-ARM ASSISTED HANG CLEAN

Stand tall with your feet shoulder-width apart and hold a dumbbell in one hand by your hip (see figure *e*). Slightly bend your knees and partially sit your hips backward so that your knees and hips are bent roughly 15 degrees (see figure *f*). Explode upward while simultaneously using your arm to pull the dumbbell up to your same-side shoulder so the dumbbell ends up in front of your shoulder with your elbow below it. As you attempt to bring the dumbbell to your shoulder, grab the back end of the dumbbell with your other hand to create some assistance and ensure the dumbbell gets where you want it (see figure *g-i*). Keep the dumbbell at your shoulder and move right into the next exercise.

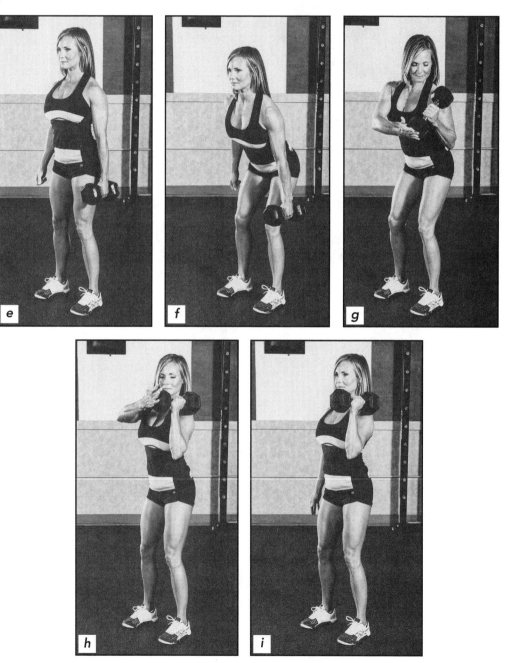

ⓘ ONE-ARM OVERHEAD PUSH PRESS

Stand tall with your feet roughly shoulder-width apart and hold a dumbbell in one hand at shoulder level with your elbow directly below the handle (see figure *j*). Slightly bend your knees (see figure *k*) and use your legs to explode upward while simultaneously pressing the dumbbell overhead (see figure *l*). Slowly lower the dumbbell to your shoulder to complete 1 rep.

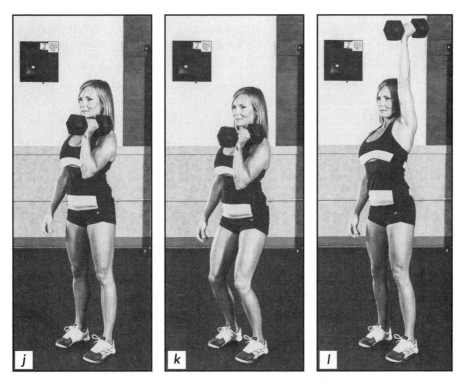

One-Arm Swing ▪
One-Arm Assisted Hang Clean ▪
One-Sided Front Squat With Dumbbell
at Shoulder ▪ One-Arm Overhead Push Press

This is another unilateral combination that enables you to use a different training stimulus than a barbell. After you've finished performing 1 rep of each of the four exercises in this combination, switch the dumbbell to the opposite hand, position your body properly for the first exercise, and repeat the sequence. You can also perform all reps on the same side first before switching sides. Following are the exercises for this combination.

1 ONE-ARM SWING

With your feet roughly hip-width apart, hold a dumbbell in one hand. Keeping your back and arm straight, drive the dumbbell between your legs as if hiking a football and hinge forward at your hips, keeping your knees bent at roughly a 15- to 20-degree angle (see figure *a*). Once your forearm comes into contact with your same-side thigh, explosively reverse the motion by simultaneously driving your hips forward and swinging the dumbbell upward to eye level to complete 1 rep (see figure *b*).

As you hinge forward, be sure that you drive your hips backward and do not allow your back to round out. Also, allowing your forearm to touch the inside of your same-side thigh at the bottom of each swing ensures that you're doing the exercise properly by emphasizing a powerful involvement of your lower-body leg and hip musculature instead of just lifting the dumbbell with your arm.

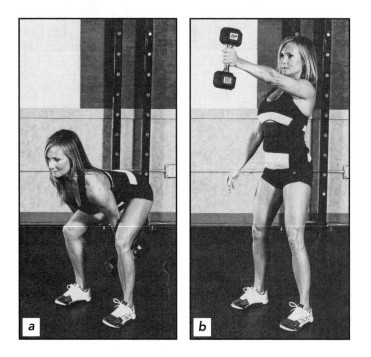

2 ONE-ARM ASSISTED HANG CLEAN

Stand tall with your feet shoulder-width apart and hold a dumbbell in one hand by your hip (see figure *c*). Slightly bend your knees and partially sit your hips backward so that your knees and hips are bent roughly 15 degrees (see figure *d*). Explode upward while simultaneously using your arm to pull the dumbbell up to your same-side shoulder so the dumbbell ends up in front of your shoulder with your elbow below it. As you attempt to bring the dumbbell to your shoulder, grab the back end of the dumbbell with your other hand to create some assistance and ensure the dumbbell gets where you want it (see figure *e-g*). Keep the dumbbell at your shoulder and move right into the next movement in this combination.

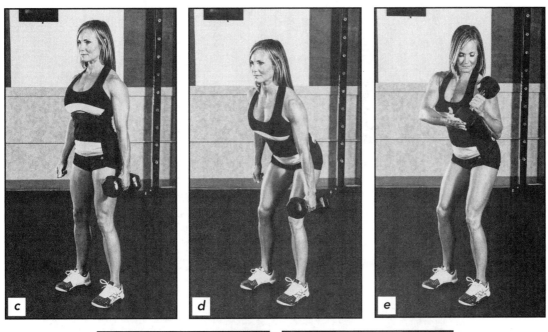

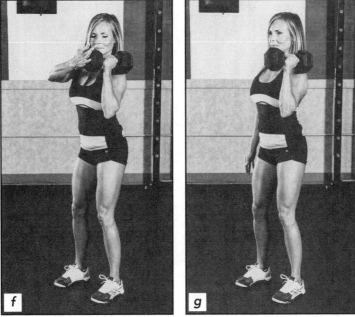

❸ ONE-SIDED FRONT SQUAT WITH DUMBBELL AT SHOULDER

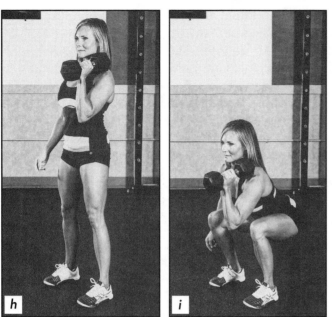

Stand tall with your feet shoulder-width apart and hold a dumbbell in one hand at shoulder level with your elbow directly below the handle (see figure *h*). While keeping your body centered, squat by bending from your knees and hips as low as you can possibly go without allowing your lower back to round out (see figure *i*). Reverse the motion and return to the tall standing position.

❹ ONE-ARM OVERHEAD PUSH PRESS

Stand tall with your feet roughly shoulder-width apart and hold a dumbbell in one hand at shoulder level with your elbow directly below the handle (see figure *j*). Slightly bend your knees (see figure *k*) and use your legs to explode upward while simultaneously pressing the dumbbell overhead (see figure *l*). Slowly lower the dumbbell to your shoulder to complete 1 rep.

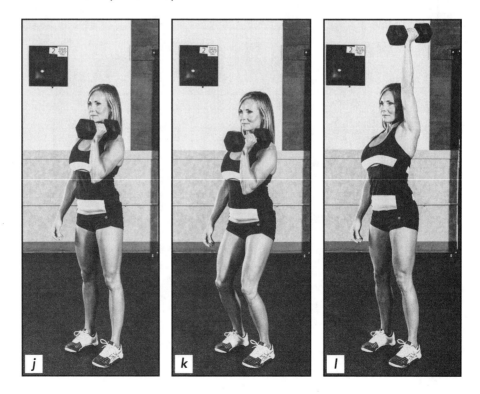

One-Arm Assisted Hang Clean ▪
One-Arm Uppercut ▪ One-Arm Swing ▪
One-Arm Burpee

This combination could be considered a hybrid exercise in that it's both a total-body and lower-body leg-oriented exercise. After you've finished performing 1 rep of each of the four exercises in this combination, switch the dumbbell to the opposite hand, position your body properly for the first exercise, and repeat the sequence. You can also perform all reps on the same side first before switching sides. Following are the exercises for this combination.

1 ONE-ARM ASSISTED HANG CLEAN

Stand tall with your feet shoulder-width apart and hold a dumbbell in one hand by your hip (see figure a). Slightly bend your knees and partially sit your hips backward so that your knees and hips are bent roughly 15 degrees (see figure b). Explode upward while simultaneously using your arm to pull the dumbbell up to your same-side shoulder so the dumbbell ends up in front of your shoulder with your elbow below it. As you attempt to bring the dumbbell to your shoulder, grab the back end of the dumbbell with your other hand to create some assistance and ensure the dumbbell gets where you want it (see figure c-e). Keep the dumbbell at your shoulder and move right into the next movement in this combination.

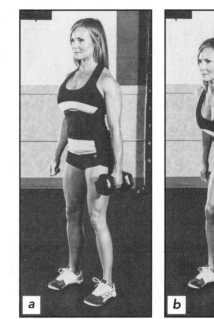

a

b

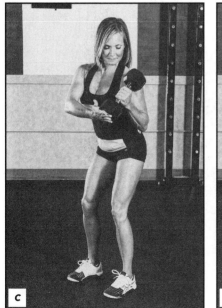

c

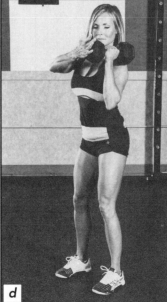

d

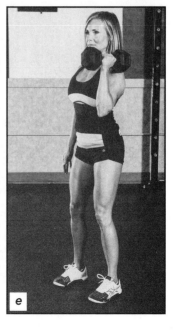

e

❷ ONE-ARM UPPERCUT

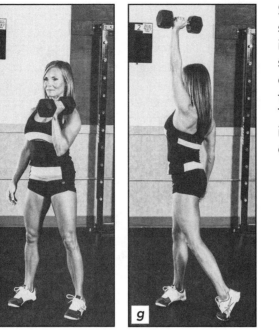

Stand tall with your feet roughly shoulder-width apart while holding a dumbbell in front of one shoulder (see figure *f*). Press the dumbbell into the air as you rotate to the opposite side (see figure *g*). To better allow your hips to rotate in this exercise, allow your heel to come off the ground as you turn.

❸ ONE-ARM SWING

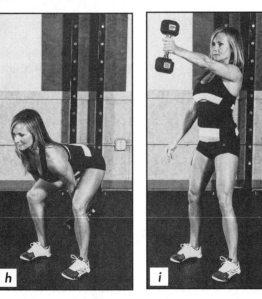

With your feet roughly hip-width apart, hold a dumbbell in one hand. Keeping your back and arm straight, drive the dumbbell between your legs as if hiking a football and hinge forward at your hips, keeping your knees bent at roughly a 15- to 20-degree angle (see figure *h*). Once your forearm comes into contact with your same-side thigh, explosively reverse the motion by simultaneously driving your hips forward and swinging the dumbbell upward to eye level to complete 1 rep (see figure *i*).

As you hinge forward, be sure that you drive your hips backward and do not allow your back to round out. Also, allowing your forearm to touch the inside of your same-side thigh at the bottom of each swing ensures that you're doing the exercise properly by emphasizing a powerful involvement of your lower-body leg and hip musculature instead of just lifting the dumbbell with your arm.

4 ONE-ARM BURPEE

With your feet slightly wider than shoulder-width apart, hold a dumbbell in one hand with your arm straight in front of your body so it's hanging between your feet (see figure *j*). With your knees slightly bent and your hips forward, place the dumbbell on the ground with your hand directly underneath your shoulder (see figure *k*) and jump your legs backward (see figure *l*) so you end up in a one-arm push-up position (see figure *m*). Make sure that your body forms one straight line and that you do not allow your hips to sag toward the floor. Jump your feet up to the dumbbell and return to the tall standing position to complete the rep (see figure *n-p*).

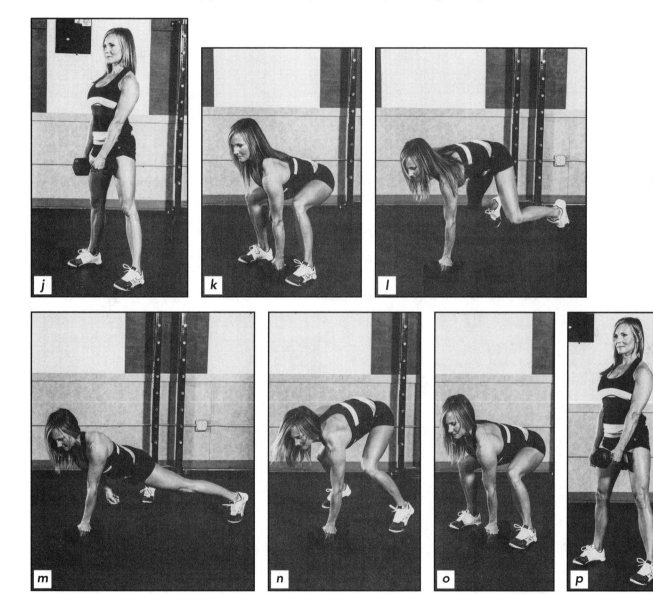

One-Arm Burpee ▪ One-Arm Assisted Hang Clean ▪ One-Sided Front Squat With Dumbbell at Shoulder ▪ One-Arm Uppercut

This is a great combination for anyone who likes to emphasize lower-body leg-oriented movements. After you've finished performing 1 rep of each of the four exercises in this combination, switch the dumbbell to the opposite hand, position your body properly for the first exercise, and repeat the sequence. You can also perform all reps on the same side first before switching sides. Following are the exercises for this combination.

1 ONE-ARM BURPEE

With your feet slightly wider than shoulder-width apart, hold a dumbbell in one hand with your arm straight in front of your body so it's hanging between your feet (see figure *a*). With your knees slightly bent and your hips forward, place the dumbbell on the ground with your hand directly underneath your shoulder (see figure *b*) and jump your legs backward (see figure *c*) so you end up in a one-arm push-up position (see figure *d*). Make sure that your body forms one straight line and that you do not allow your hips to sag toward the floor. Jump your feet up to the dumbbell (see figures *e* and *f*) and return to the tall standing position to complete the rep.

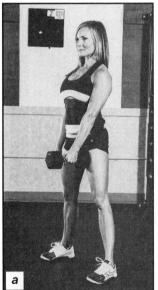

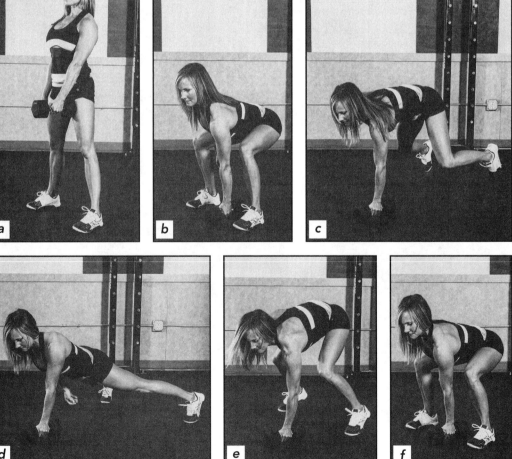

2 ONE-ARM ASSISTED HANG CLEAN

Stand tall with your feet shoulder-width apart and hold a dumbbell in one hand by your hip (see figure g). Slightly bend your knees and partially sit your hips backward so that your knees and hips are bent roughly 15 degrees (see figure h). Explode upward while simultaneously using your arm to pull the dumbbell up to your same-side shoulder so the dumbbell ends up in front of your shoulder with your elbow below it. As you attempt to bring the dumbbell to your shoulder, grab the back end of the dumbbell with your other hand to create some assistance and ensure the dumbbell gets where you want it (see figure i-k). Keep the dumbbell at your shoulder and move right into the next movement in this combination.

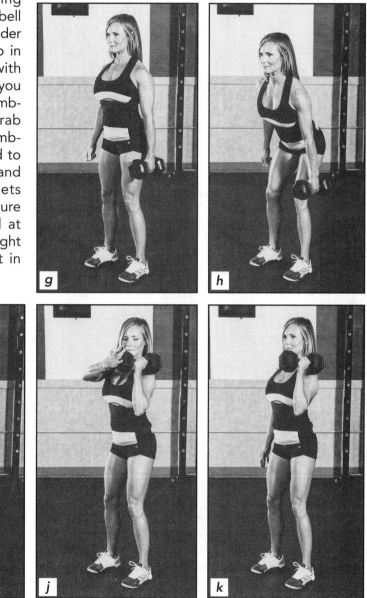

3 ONE-SIDED FRONT SQUAT WITH DUMBBELL AT SHOULDER

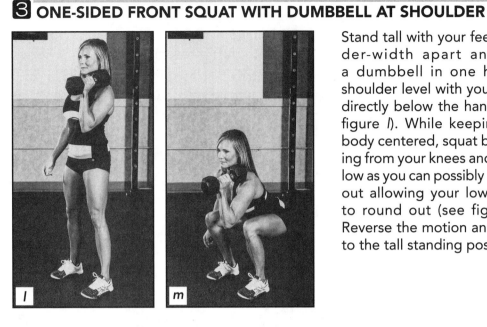

Stand tall with your feet shoulder-width apart and hold a dumbbell in one hand at shoulder level with your elbow directly below the handle (see figure *l*). While keeping your body centered, squat by bending from your knees and hips as low as you can possibly go without allowing your lower back to round out (see figure *m*). Reverse the motion and return to the tall standing position.

4 ONE-ARM UPPERCUT

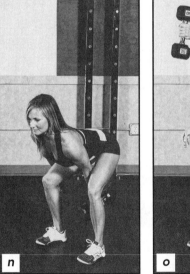
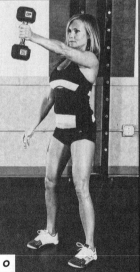

Stand tall with your feet roughly shoulder-width apart while holding a dumbbell in front of one shoulder (see figure *n*). Press the dumbbell into the air as you rotate to the opposite side (see figure *o*). To better allow your hips to rotate in this exercise, allow your heel to come off the ground as you turn.

Squat and Press ▪ Two-Arm Swing ▪ Down Burpee ▪ Push-Up ▪ Plank Row ▪ Up Burpee

This is the first bilateral combination in the dumbbell category, meaning that it uses two dumbbells, one in each hand. This combination also adds a new dimension to the burpee exercise, as you'll see in the step-by-step descriptions. After you've finished performing 1 rep of each of the four exercises in this complex, position your body properly to start the first exercise and repeat the sequence. Following are the exercises in this combination.

1 SQUAT AND PRESS

Stand tall with your feet shoulder-width apart and hold a dumbbell in each hand at your shoulders with your elbows directly underneath the handles (see figure a). Squat as low as you can by bending your knees and sitting your hips back without allowing your heels to rise off the floor or your lower back to round out (see figure b). Reverse the motion by simultaneously standing up and pressing the dumbbells overhead so that your knees and arms straighten at roughly the same time (see figure c).

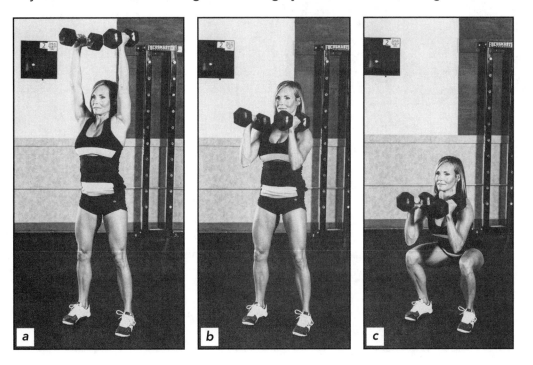

❷ TWO-ARM SWING

With your feet roughly hip-width apart, hold a dumbbell in each hand. Keeping your back and arms straight, drive the dumbbells between your legs as if hiking a football and hinge forward at your hips, keeping your knees bent at roughly a 15- to 20-degree angle (see figure d). Once your forearms come into contact with your thighs, explosively reverse the motion by simultaneously driving your hips forward and swinging

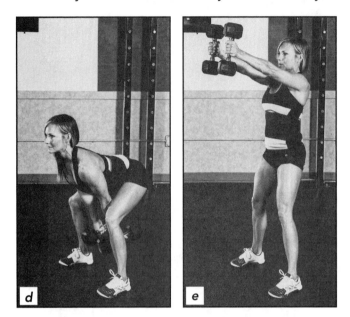

the dumbbells upward to eye level to complete 1 rep (see figure e).

As you hinge forward, be sure that you drive your hips backward and do not allow your back to round out. Also, allow your forearms to touch the insides of your thighs at the bottom of each swing. Use your hips to powerfully drive your arms forward off your thighs to swing the dumbbells up on each rep. This ensures that you're doing the exercise properly by emphasizing a powerful involvement of your lower-body leg and hip musculature instead of just lifting the dumbbell with your arms.

❸ DOWN BURPEE

Stand with your feet wider than shoulder-width apart and hold dumbbells in front of your hips with your arms straight so they are hanging in between your feet. Bend your knees and hinge forward at your hips to place the dumbbells on the floor between your feet directly under each shoulder (see figure f). Jump your feet backward so you end up in push-up position with your body forming a straight line, and do not allow your hips to sag toward the floor (see figure g). Remain in this position and move to the next exercise.

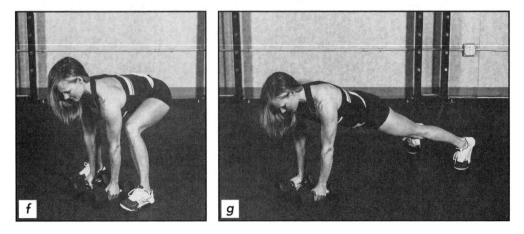

4 PUSH-UP

With dumbbells directly under your shoulders, place one hand on the handle of each dumbbell (see figure *h*). Perform a push-up by lowering your body to the floor while keeping your elbows directly above your wrists the entire time (see figure *i*). Once your ribs come in contact with the dumbbells, reverse the motion by pushing your body up. Be sure you do not allow your head or hips to sag toward the floor at any time.

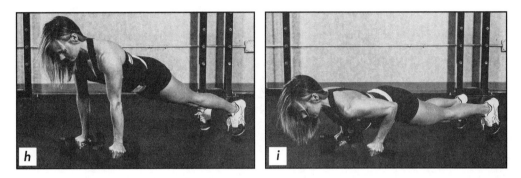

5 PLANK ROW

While in the push-up plank position with each hand holding the handle of each dumbbell (see figure *j*), row one dumbbell up into your body until it touches the same-side ribs (see figure *k*). Slowly lower the dumbbell to the floor and row the other dumbbell in the same manner. While rowing the dumbbells, be sure your torso remains as stable as possible and your hips do not rotate at any time.

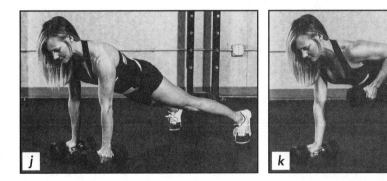

6 UP BURPEE

While in the push-up plank position with each hand holding the handle of each dumbbell, jump your feet up so that they are on each side of the dumbbells (see figure *l*). Then simply stand up tall (see figure *m*).

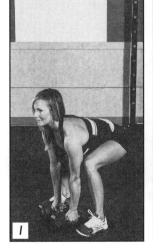
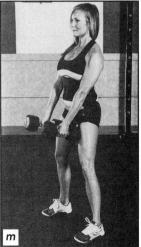

Squat Jump ▪ Down Burpee ▪ T-Roll Push-Up ▪ Up Burpee

This combination also involves two dumbbells, and it's great for someone who's looking to challenge the muscles of the torso, especially the anterior abdominal muscles. After you've finished performing 1 rep of each of the four exercises in this combination, position your body properly for the first exercise, and repeat the sequence. Following are the exercises in this combination.

1 SQUAT JUMP

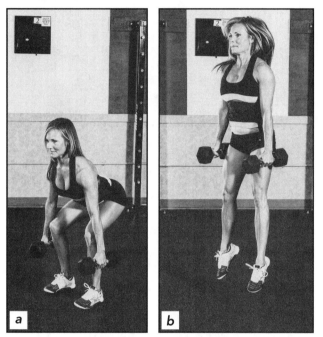

With your feet roughly shoulder-width apart, stand tall holding one dumbbell in each hand outside your hips and squat so that your thighs are parallel or slightly below parallel with the floor, making sure you do not allow your lower back to round out (see figure a). Explode up by extending your legs and jumping into the air (see figure b). Land as lightly and as quietly as possible into a squat position. Make sure that each time you squat down your knees remain in the same line as your toes; your knees should not come toward one another at any time.

2 DOWN BURPEE

Stand with your feet wider than shoulder-width apart and hold dumbbells in front of your hips with your arms straight so they are hanging in between your feet. Bend your knees and hinge forward at your hips to place the dumbbells on the floor between your feet directly under each shoulder (see figure c). Jump your feet backward so you end up in push-up position with your body forming a straight line, and do not allow your hips to sag toward the floor (see figure d).

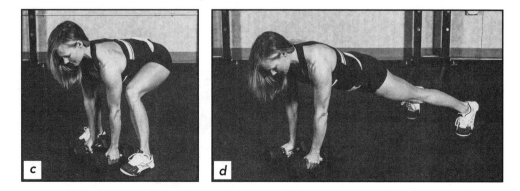

❸ T-ROLL PUSH-UP

While in a push-up plank position with your hands on the handles of the dumbbells, which are directly under your shoulders, perform a push-up by lowering your body to the floor while keeping your elbows directly above your wrists the entire time (see figure *e*). Once your ribs come in contact with the dumbbells, reverse the motion by pushing your body up (see figure *f*). At the top of each repetition, perform a T-roll by rotating your entire body to one side, rolling to the sides of your feet and simultaneously reaching your top arm to the sky so that your body forms the letter *T* (see figure *g*). Reverse the motion by rolling to the other side and reaching your other arm toward the sky. Then come back to the middle and assume the push-up plank position. Be sure you do not allow your head or hips to sag toward the floor at any time.

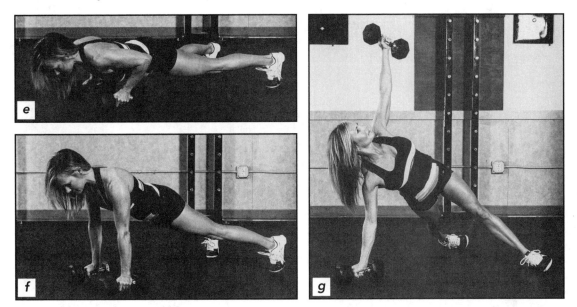

❹ UP BURPEE

While in the push-up plank position with each hand holding the handle of each dumbbell, jump your feet up so that they are on each side of the dumbbells (see figure *h*). Then simply stand up tall (see figure *i*).

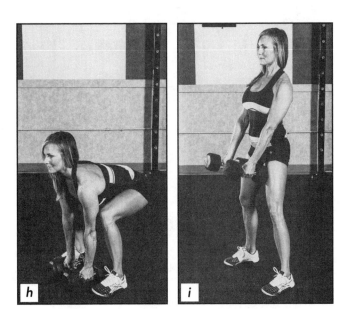

Turkish Get-Up

Although the Turkish get-up has a single name, it is truly a combination of several exercises that can be done while holding a dumbbell (or kettlebell). If you've never tried the Turkish get-up, get ready for an exercise that's unlike any other.

Lie supine on the floor, holding a dumbbell (or kettlebell) in your left hand. Reach your arm toward the sky directly above your shoulder and bend your left knee (see figure *a*). Roll to your right elbow, keeping your left arm stable (see figure *b*). Then extend your right elbow to sit up (see figure *c*). Raise your hips into the air (see figure *d*) and slide your right leg underneath your body (see figure *e*), placing your right knee on the floor while continuing to keep your left arm straight and stable (see figure *f*). Then raise your torso so that it's perpendicular to the floor (see figure *g*). Finally, stand up out of the half-kneeling position (see figure *h*). Then slowly reverse each motion step by step until you're in the starting position in order to complete 1 rep. Repeat on the other side. Note that you can switch hands after each rep or switch sides every two, three, or four reps and so on—whatever you feel is needed to maintain optimal intensity and control when performing the exercise.

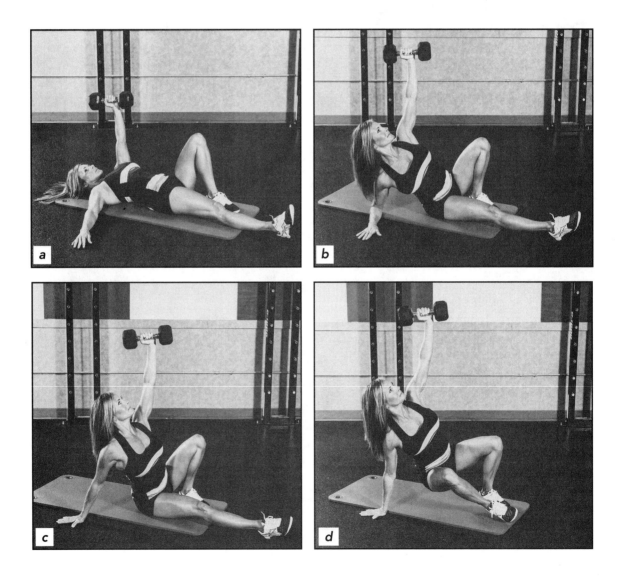

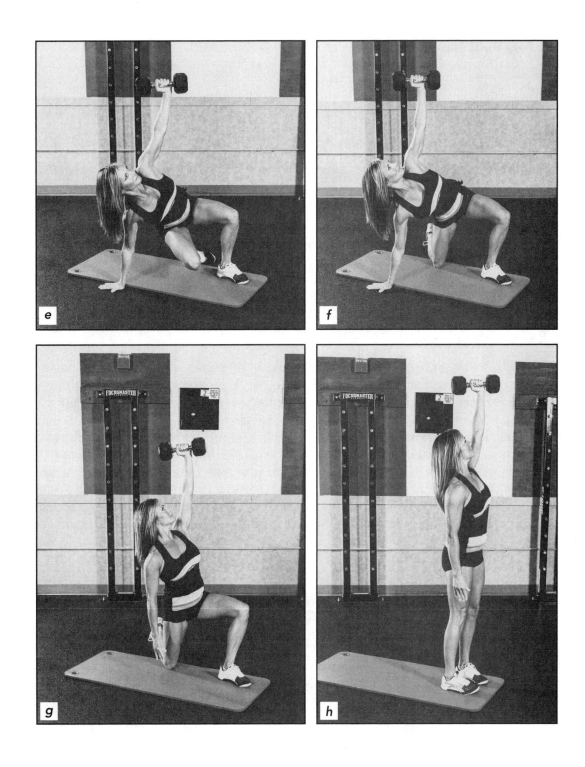

Kettlebell Exercises

Kettlebells are a natural and effective option for performing combinations because many kettlebell moves flow together nicely. That said, it takes some practice to get comfortable using kettlebells. When using kettlebells in a gym setting, be sure to have plenty of space around you and be aware of your surroundings. Your fellow gym members may not be used to the swinging actions and may walk by close enough to get hit.

Two-Arm Swing ▪ Two-Arm Swing Clean ▪ Front Squat ▪ Two-Arm Overhead Push Press

This combination involves two kettlebells and incorporates four primary kettlebell exercises. Following are the exercises for this combination.

1 TWO-ARM SWING

With your feet roughly hip-width apart, hold a kettlebell in each hand. Keeping your back and arms straight, drive the kettlebells between your legs as if hiking a football and hinge forward at your hips, keeping your knees bent at roughly a 15- to 20-degree angle (see figure a). Once your forearms come into contact with your thighs, explosively reverse the motion by simultaneously driving your hips forward and swinging the kettlebells upward to eye level to complete 1 rep (see figure b).

As you hinge forward, be sure that you drive your hips backward and do not allow your back to round out. Also, allow your forearms to touch the insides of your thighs at the bottom of each swing. Use your hips to powerfully drive your arms forward off your thighs to swing the kettlebells back up on each rep. This ensures that you're doing the exercise properly by emphasizing a powerful involvement of your lower-body leg and hip musculature instead of just lifting the kettlebells with your arms.

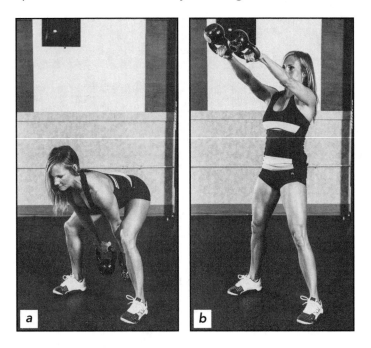

2 TWO-ARM SWING CLEAN

Stand with your feet wider than shoulder-width apart and hold a kettlebell in each hand. Slightly bend your knees and hinge at your hips to allow the kettlebells to swing between your legs (see figure c). Quickly reverse this motion by driving your hips forward and moving your arms upward (see figure d). As the kettlebells move toward the sky, quickly flip your elbows underneath them and soften your body to accept the kettlebells moving into your body, creating as much of a cushion as you can (see figure e and f). In other words, as the kettlebells come up to your chest, imagine that they're eggs that you do not want to break, absorbing them as gently as possible.

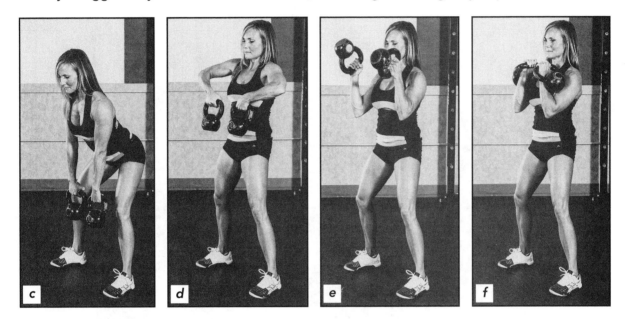

3 FRONT SQUAT

With your feet slightly wider than shoulder-width apart and toes turned out 10 to 15 degrees, hold the kettlebells in front of you, resting them on the top of your chest and forearms (see figure g). Your hands should be closer to the center of your chest and your elbows should be close to the sides of your body, pointing down like a triangle. Be sure to stay tall and lift your chest to create a rack for the kettlebells instead of trying to hold them up using only your arms. Bend at your knees and hips and lower your body toward the floor as low as you can possibly go (see figure h). Your heels should not lift off the ground and your lower back should not lose its arch. Also, be sure to keep your knees wide and tracking in the same direction as your toes and do not allow your knees to drop in toward the midline of your body. Once you've gone as deep as you can control in the squat, reverse the motion and stand up.

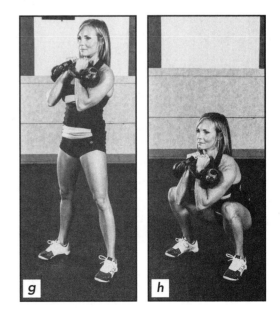

4 TWO-ARM OVERHEAD PUSH PRESS

Stand with your feet shoulder-width apart, holding the kettlebells with your hands just outside shoulder-width apart with the kettlebells resting on the top of your chest and forearms (see figure *i*). Your hands should be closer to the center of your chest and your elbows should be pointing down like a triangle. Slightly bend your knees (see figure *j*) and then quickly reverse the motion, exploding into the kettlebells by pressing them overhead using both your arms and legs in a coordinated fashion, finishing with your palms facing each other (see figure *k*). Once the kettlebells are completely overhead, slowly reverse the motion by lowering them to the starting position.

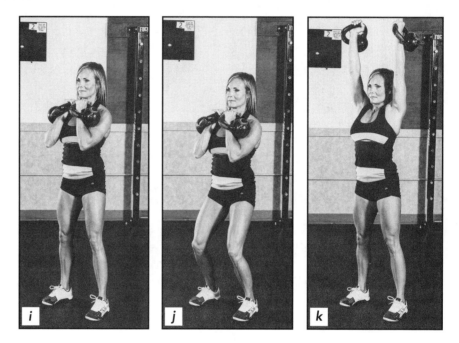

One-Arm Swing ▪ One-Arm Swing Clean
One-Sided Front Squat ▪
One-Arm Overhead Push Press

This combination is performed exactly the same as the previous combination, except all the exercises are done unilaterally, using the same arm to complete each move. This is a great complex for someone who enjoys using kettlebells and is also interested in the additional demand on the torso that is created by unilateral exercises. Following are the exercises for this combination.

1 ONE-ARM SWING

With your feet roughly hip-width apart, hold a kettlebell in one hand with your arm straight. Keeping your back and arm straight, drive the kettlebell between your legs as if hiking a football and hinge forward at your hips, keeping your knees bent at roughly a 15- to 20-degree angle (see figure *a*). Once your forearm comes into contact with your thigh, explosively reverse the motion by simultaneously driving your hips forward and swinging the kettlebell upward to eye level (see figure *b*).

As you hinge forward, be sure that you drive your hips backward and do not allow your back to round out. Also, by allowing your forearm to touch the inside of your thigh at the bottom of each swing, you use your hips to powerfully drive your arm forward off your thigh to swing the kettlebell up on each rep. This ensures that you're doing the kettlebell swing properly by emphasizing a powerful involvement of your lower-body leg and hip musculature instead of just lifting the kettlebell with your arm.

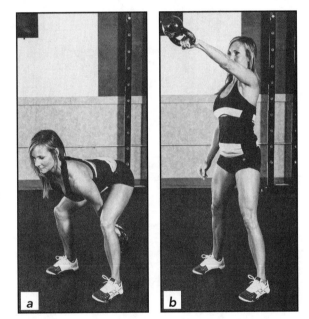

❷ ONE-ARM SWING CLEAN

Stand with your feet wider than shoulder-width apart and hold a kettlebell in one hand. Slightly bend your knees and hinge at your hips to allow the kettlebell to swing between your legs (see figure c). Quickly reverse this motion by driving your hips forward and your arm upward (see figure d). As the kettlebell moves toward the sky, quickly flip your elbow underneath it and soften your body to accept the kettlebell moving into your body, creating as much of a cushion as you can (see figure e). In other words, as the kettlebell comes up to your chest, imagine it's an egg that you do not want to break, absorbing it as gently as possible.

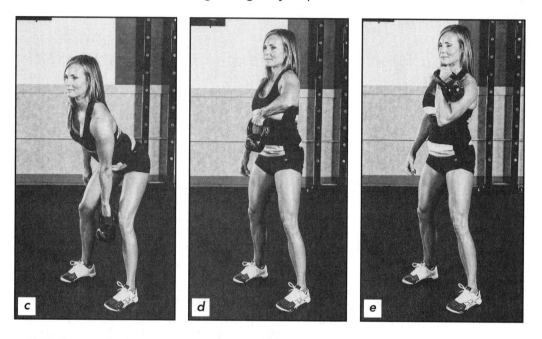

❸ ONE-SIDED FRONT SQUAT

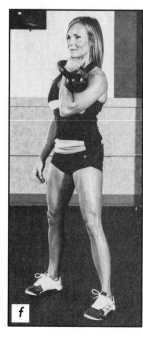
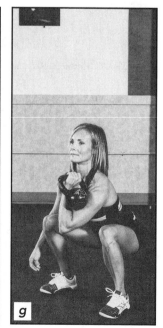

With your feet slightly wider than shoulder-width apart and toes turned out 10 to 15 degrees, hold a kettlebell in front of you, resting it on the top of your chest and forearm on the side you are holding the kettlebell (see figure f). Your hand should be closer to the center of your chest and your elbow should be pointing down like a triangle. Be sure to stay tall and lift your chest to create a rack for the kettlebell instead of trying to hold it up using only your arm. Bend at your knees and hips and lower your body toward the floor as low as you can possibly go (see figure g). Your heels should not lift off the ground and your lower back should not lose its arch.

Also, be sure to keep your knees wide and tracking in the same direction as your toes and do not allow your knees to drop in toward the midline of your body. Once you've gone as deep as you can control in the squat, reverse the motion and stand up.

4 ONE-ARM OVERHEAD PUSH PRESS

Stand with your feet shoulder-width apart and hold a kettlebell on the top of your chest and forearm (see figure *h*). Your hand should be closer to the center of your chest and your elbow should be pointing down like the side of a triangle. Slightly bend your knees (see figure *i*) and then quickly reverse the motion, exploding into the kettlebell by pressing it overhead using both your arm and legs in a coordinated fashion (see figure *j*). Once the kettlebell is completely overhead, slowly reverse the motion by lowering it to the starting position.

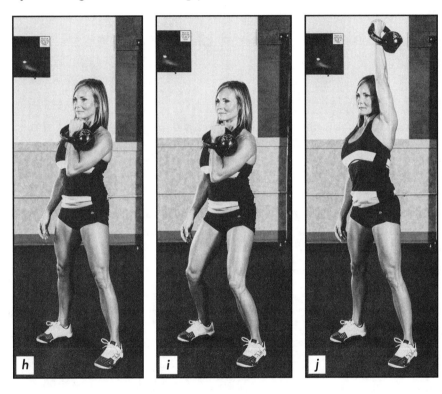

Core-Bar Exercises

The core bar is a unilaterally loaded bar that can be loaded by either using weight plates or attaching it to a cable column or resistance band. What makes the core bar unique is that it offers reciprocal movement training—while one side is pushing, the other side is pulling, and vice versa. This type of reciprocal action happens in a range of functional activities from walking to throwing a punch—while one side goes forward, the other side is going in the opposite direction. In short, barbells and two-arm kettlebell and dumbbell exercises offer bilateral movements. Single-arm kettlebell and dumbbell exercises offer unilateral movements. And the core bar offers the unique opportunity to load reciprocal movements. In addition, the core bar offers a few exercises that you just can't do with other types of exercise equipment.

Shovel Clean ▪ Liberty Press

1 SHOVEL CLEAN

Stand with your feet shoulder-width apart. With your left hand, hold the bottom of the core bar in an overhand grip, and with your right hand, hold higher up on the bar (closer to the weighted end) with an underhand grip. The weighted end of the core bar faces away from you. Squat down so the nonweighted end of the core bar is resting on top of your left thigh and your left hand is to the side of your left hip (see figure a). Push down with your left hand while simultaneously lifting up with your right hand and lift the core bar toward your right shoulder as if shoveling something over your right shoulder (see figure b and c).

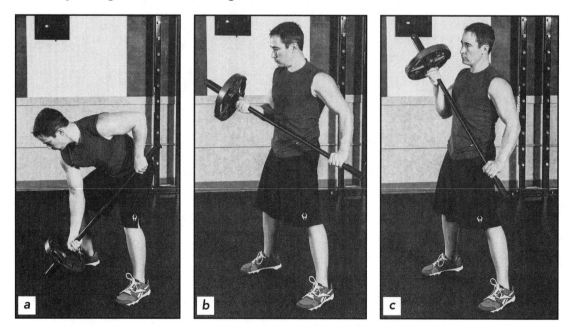

❷ LIBERTY PRESS

Stand with your feet roughly shoulder-width apart. Hold the core bar at your right shoulder with your left hand at the bottom, palm facing toward your body, while your right hand is at the top underneath the weight plates, also facing your body (see figure *d*). Slightly bend your knees and simultaneously extend your legs as you push the core bar toward the sky, keeping it vertical (see figure *e*). Slowly lower the bar to where you started so you end up in position ready to perform the shovel clean with the end of the bar back down to the floor and the bottom handle back to the top of your left thigh to start the next repetition.

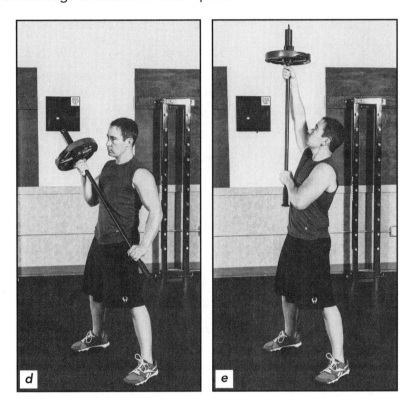

The metabolic combinations in this chapter all have one thing in common: Each exercise is strategically placed in an order that allows you to smoothly transition into the exercise that follows. This makes these combinations not only easier to memorize but also more effective, because they allow you to get a lot of high-quality exercise done while integrating a wide variety of movements into a short amount of time. The complexes that are described in the following chapter share the same positive qualities.

chapter 6

Complexes

A complex is a series of strength training exercises that are each performed for multiple reps using the same piece of equipment. Like the metabolic strength training combinations covered in the previous chapter, these complexes also involve performing multiple strength training exercises back to back with a seamless flow from one exercise to the next, which helps makes them easy to memorize. However, unlike combinations, complexes involve performing several reps (rep clusters) of an exercise within a given complex before moving on to the next exercise in the complex without resting in between.

COMPLEX TRAINING

A complex is a full-body circuit where all of the stations involve one piece of equipment, which is helpful in a crowded gym with lots of people all trying to use the same equipment. You can string together any number of exercises to form a complex. The more exercises used, the more intense the complex becomes due to the increased volume.

The weight load used to perform these complexes is lighter than the load used in the circuits and combinations, because complexes are performed at a faster pace and a higher volume than circuits and combinations. When performing a complex, the goal is to move the weight (i.e., perform each rep) at a fast pace without losing control of the weight or your own body positioning. In other words, you want to move fast (to keep the intensity high) without rushing; it's not a race and you don't want to get sloppy. There are two ways to boost the intensity of your workouts and to recruit maximal motor units: move something heavy or move fast. The metabolic strength training protocols in this book use both methods to ensure your workouts are well rounded and maximally effective—you move fast with lighter loads when performing complexes, and you lift heavier loads with less speed when doing circuits and combinations.

Using the same strategy as the circuits covered in chapter 4, each complex described in this chapter includes these basic movement patterns:

- Upper-body pushing movement
- Upper-body pulling movement
- Lower-body leg-oriented movement (e.g., squats)
- Lower-body hip-oriented movement (e.g., deadlifts)

When you perform each of these movement patterns, you hit all the muscle groups of the body in some fashion. This includes your core musculature, because those muscles work every time you have to maintain a strong and stable body position, which is required to perform any of the complexes featured in this chapter. And of course, we've already established that more muscles worked equals more calories burned—both during your workout and for many hours afterward.

COMPLEXES

The following metabolic strength training complexes incorporate four exercises or more, covering some of the movement patterns several times with different exercises within a given complex. For each complex, you perform a cluster of reps for an exercise before moving to the next exercise within the same complex.

Before learning how to perform a variety of complexes, you need to know the parameters for using them:

- Use the heaviest load possible to complete the reps while moving quickly with good control through the complex.

- Perform 6 to 15 reps per exercise within a given complex and 2 to 5 sets per complex.

- There is no rest between exercises within a given complex (unless you need to take a quick breath). However, you should rest from 90 seconds to 3 minutes between complexes (i.e., after completing a full round of a complex).

- If performing a unilateral complex (working one side at a time), rest 30 to 90 seconds between sides, and rest 2 to 3 minutes after completing a full round on each side.

It is recommended that you use a *higher* number of repetitions for the easier exercises (the ones you're strongest at performing) within a complex and use a *lower* number of repetitions for the most difficult exercises (the ones you're weakest at performing). To ensure consistent progression, add load, add repetitions, or reduce rest time between complexes.

Following are some bilateral and unilateral metabolic complexes. As you'll see, a few of the sequences from the combinations provided in the previous chapter can also be used as a complex.

Barbell Complexes

The barbell is not only a great tool for gaining strength and for putting together exercise combinations, it's also effective for building metabolic strength training complexes that are sure have your muscles pumping and your heart pounding. Here are various metabolic strength training complexes that show you new ways to use an old training tool and apply classic, battle-tested barbell exercises.

Reverse Lunge ■ Overhead Push Press ■ Wide-Grip Bent-Over Row ■ Wide-Grip Romanian Deadlift

1 REVERSE LUNGE

Stand tall with your feet hip-width apart and a barbell across your shoulders behind your head (see figure *a*). Step backward with one foot and drop your body so your knee lightly touches the floor (see figure *b*). Reverse the movement by coming out of the lunge and bringing the same foot forward so that you are back to your starting position. Perform the same movement on the opposite leg.

Note: After performing the last repetition of the reverse lunge, use your legs and arms in a coordinated fashion to lift the barbell off the back of your shoulders to the front of your body to begin the overhead push press.

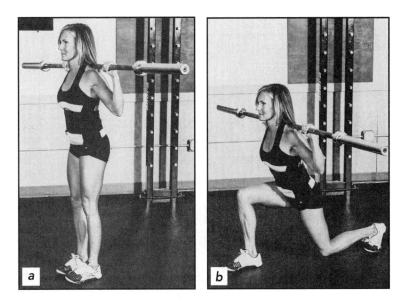

2 OVERHEAD PUSH PRESS

Stand with your feet shoulder-width apart and hold the barbell with your hands just outside shoulder-width apart (see figure *c*). Slightly bend your knees (see figure *d*) and then quickly reverse the motion, exploding into the bar and driving the barbell overhead using both your arms and legs in a coordinated fashion (see figure *e*). Once the bar is completely overhead, slowly lower the barbell back down to complete 1 full repetition.

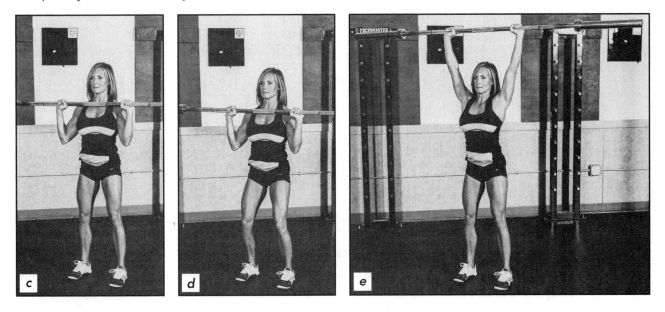

❸ WIDE-GRIP BENT-OVER ROW

Stand with your feet shoulder-width apart and hold a barbell with your hands roughly 12 inches outside each hip. Bend over at your hips, keeping your back straight so that your torso is parallel to the floor and keeping your knees bent 15 to 20 degrees (see figure *f*). Row the bar into the middle of your torso between your chest and your belly button (see figure *g*). Slowly lower the bar without allowing it to contact the floor until the set is completed.

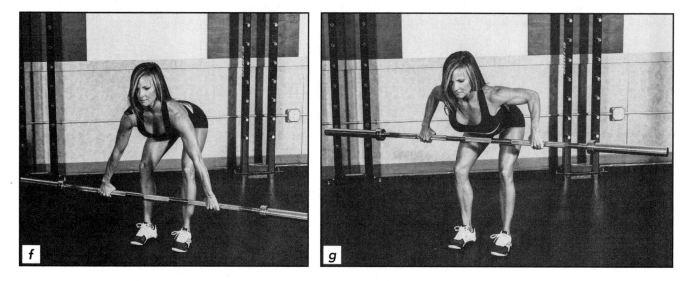

❹ WIDE-GRIP ROMANIAN DEADLIFT

Stand with your feet shoulder-width apart and hold a barbell in front of your thighs with your arms straight and your hands placed on the bar roughly 12 inches outside each hip (see figure *h*). Keeping your back straight, hinge at your hips and bend forward toward the floor, keeping your knees bent at roughly a 15- to 20-degree angle (see figure *i*). As you hinge forward, drive your hips backward and do not allow your back to round out.

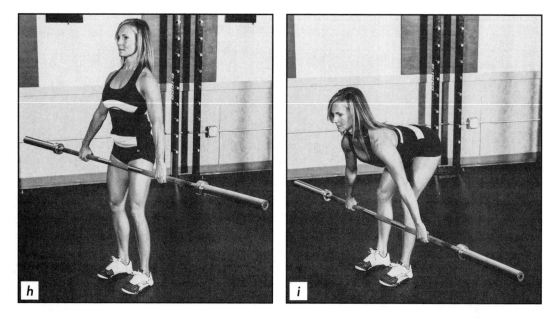

Bent-Over Row ▪ Romanian Deadlift ▪ Hang Clean ▪ Overhead Push Press ▪ Front Squat

1 BENT-OVER ROW

Stand with your feet roughly hip-width apart. Hold the barbell using an underhand grip, keeping your hands just outside shoulder-width apart. Bend over at your hips, keeping your back straight so that your torso is parallel to the floor and your knees are bent 15 to 20 degrees (see figure *a*). Row the bar into the middle of your torso between your chest and your belly button (see figure *b*). Slowly lower the bar without allowing the barbell to touch the ground. You can also perform bent-over rows by using an overhand grip, which many people find to be a less strong gripping option.

Note: After finishing your bent-over rows, place the barbell on the floor and switch to an overhand grip to perform the Romanian deadlift and the rest of the exercises in this combination.

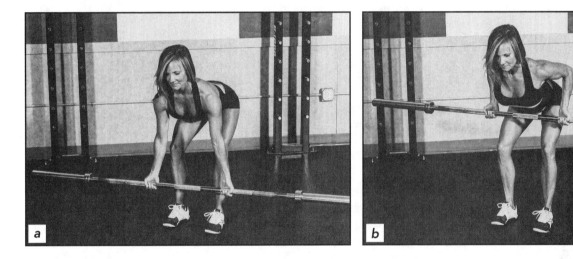

2 ROMANIAN DEADLIFT

Stand tall with your feet hip-width apart, holding a barbell in front of your thighs with your arms straight (see figure *c*). Keeping your back straight, hinge at your hips and bend forward toward the floor, keeping your knees bent at a 15- to 20-degree angle (see figure *d*). As you hinge forward, drive your hips backward and do not allow your back to round out. Once your torso is roughly parallel to the floor or the weight plates lightly tap the floor, drive your hips forward toward the barbell, reversing the motion to stand tall again.

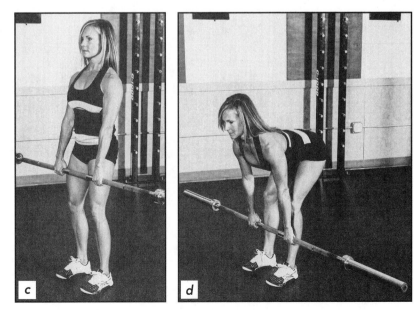

❸ HANG CLEAN

Stand with your feet shoulder-width apart and hold a barbell with your hands just outside shoulder-width apart. Slightly hinge at your hips, keeping the bar against your thighs (see figure *e*), and explode your hips into the bar as you simultaneously pull the bar upward (see figure *f*). Once the bar reaches shoulder level (see figure *g*), quickly flip your elbows underneath the bar to catch it at the top of your chest (see figure *h*).

Note: After performing your last hang clean repetition, hold the barbell at the top of the position, setting up to begin the overhead push press.

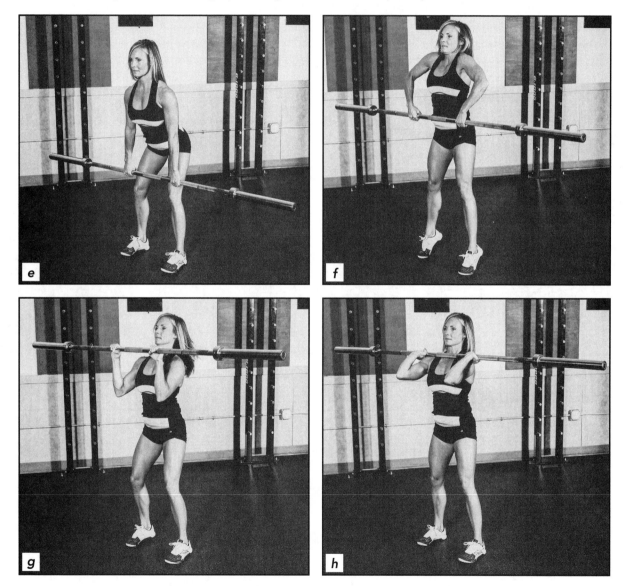

4 OVERHEAD PUSH PRESS

Stand with your feet shoulder-width apart and hold the barbell with your hands just outside shoulder-width apart (see figure *i*). Slightly bend your knees (see figure *j*) and then quickly reverse the motion, exploding into the bar and driving it overhead using both your arms and legs in a coordinated fashion (see figure *k*). Once the bar is completely overhead, slowly lower the barbell back down to complete 1 full repetition.

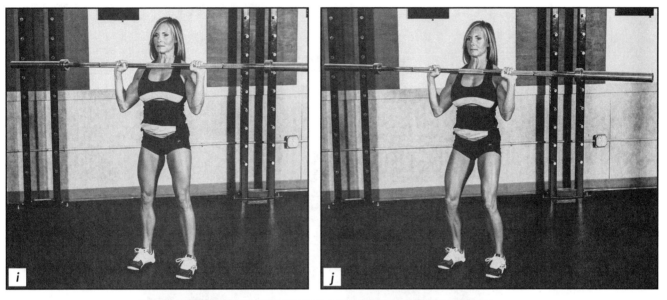

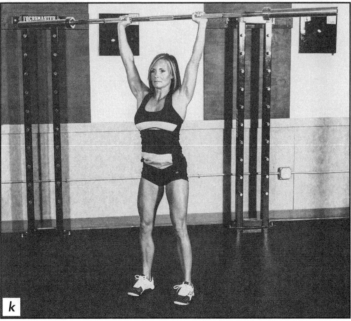

5 FRONT SQUAT

With the bar resting on the top of your chest and your elbows pointing straight out in front of you so they are parallel to the floor (see figure *l*), perform a squat, dropping as low as you possibly can while maintaining optimal control of your knee and spinal alignment (see figure *m*). Reverse the motion by standing up to begin the next repetition of this complex.

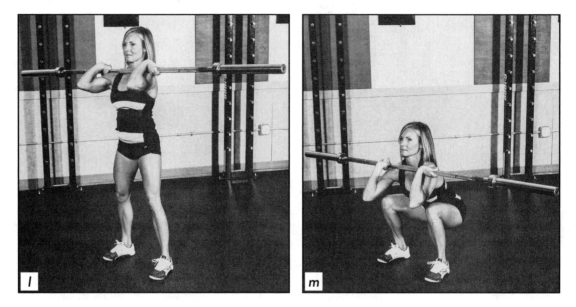

Romanian Deadlift ▪ Hang Clean ▪ Front Squat ▪ Overhead Push Press ▪ Good Morning ▪ Reverse Lunge ▪ Barbell Calf Raise

1 ROMANIAN DEADLIFT

Stand tall with your feet hip-width apart, holding a barbell in front of your thighs with your arms straight (see figure a). Keeping your back straight, hinge at your hips and bend forward toward the floor, keeping your knees bent at a 15- to 20-degree angle (see figure b). As you hinge forward, drive your hips backward and do not allow your back to round out. Once your torso is roughly parallel to the floor or the weight plates lightly tap the floor, drive your hips forward toward the barbell, reversing the motion to stand tall again.

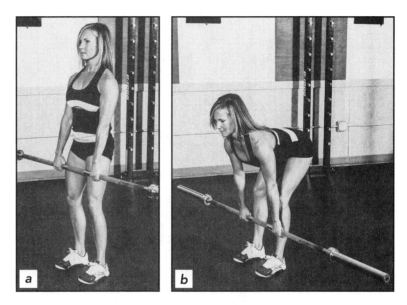

2 HANG CLEAN

Stand with your feet shoulder-width apart and hold a barbell with your hands just outside shoulder-width apart. Slightly hinge at your hips, keeping the bar against your thighs (see figure c), and explode your hips into the bar as you simultaneously pull the bar upward (see figure d). Once the bar reaches shoulder level (see figure e), quickly flip your elbows underneath the bar to catch it at the top of your chest (see figure f).

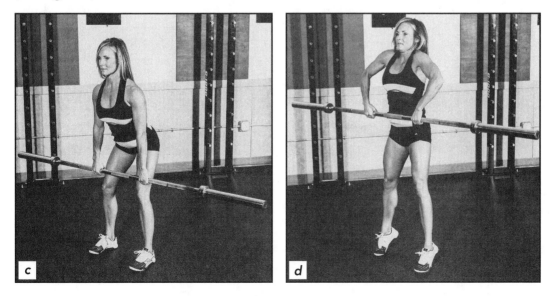

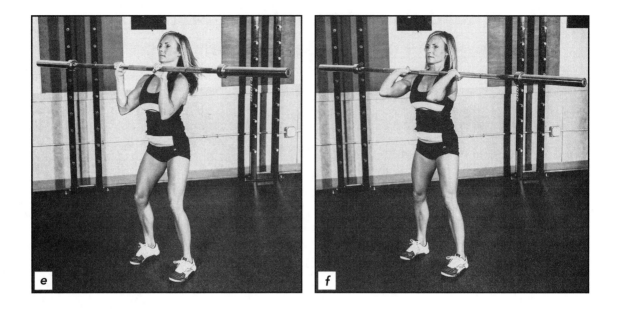

3 FRONT SQUAT

With the bar resting on the top of your chest and your elbows pointing straight out in front of you so they are parallel to the floor (see figure g), perform a squat, dropping as low as you possibly can while maintaining optimal control of your knee and spinal alignment (see figure h). Reverse the motion by standing up to begin the next repetition of this complex.

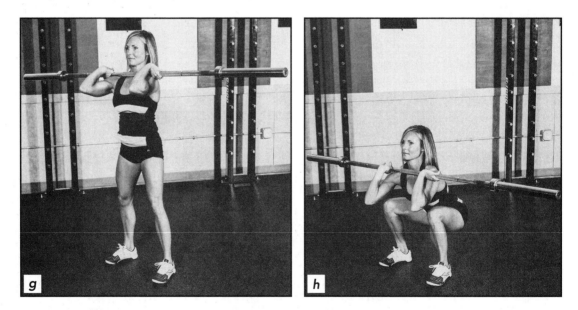

4 OVERHEAD PUSH PRESS

Stand with your feet shoulder-width apart and hold the barbell with your hands just outside shoulder-width apart (see figure *i*). Slightly bend your knees (see figure *j*) and then quickly reverse the motion, exploding into the bar and driving it overhead using both your arms and legs in a coordinated fashion (see figure *k*). Once the bar is completely overhead, slowly lower the barbell back down to complete 1 full repetition.

Note: After performing your last overhead push press, lower the barbell behind your head and place it across your shoulders to set up for the next exercise, good morning.

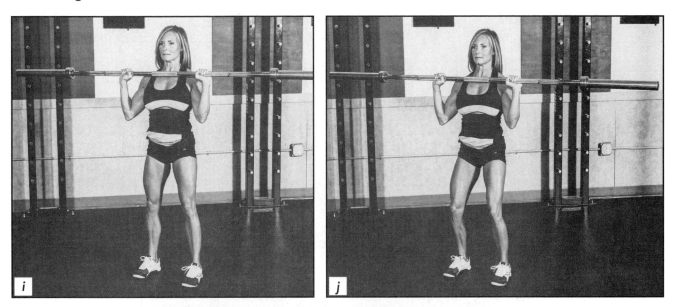

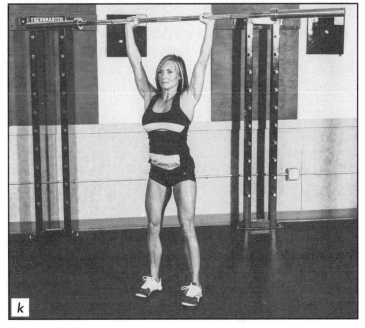

5 GOOD MORNING

Stand tall with your feet hip-width apart and place a barbell across your shoulders behind your head (see figure *l*). Keeping your back straight, hinge at your hips and bend forward toward the floor, keeping your knees bent at roughly a 15- to 20-degree angle (see figure *m*). As you hinge forward, drive your hips backward and do not allow your back to round out. Once your torso is roughly parallel to the floor, drive your hips forward toward the barbell, reversing the motion to stand tall again and complete 1 rep.

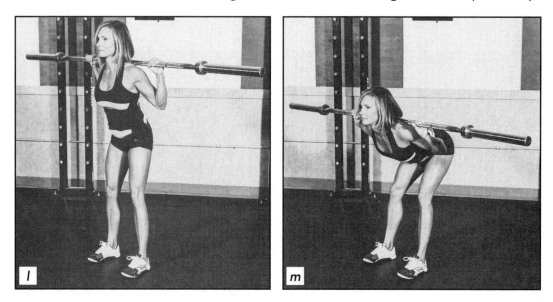

6 REVERSE LUNGE

Stand tall with your feet hip-width apart and a barbell across your shoulders behind your head (see figure *n*). Step backward with one foot and drop your body so your knee lightly touches the floor (see figure *o*). Reverse the movement by coming out of the lunge and bringing the same foot forward so that you are back to your starting position. Perform the same movement on the opposite leg.

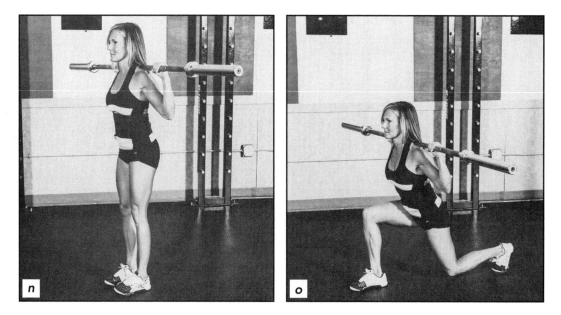

7 BARBELL CALF RAISE

Stand tall with your feet hip-width apart and place a barbell across the top of your shoulders behind your head (see figure p). Simultaneously push your toes into the ground and lift your heels as high as you can off the floor to end up on the balls of your feet (see figure q). Slowly lower yourself until your heels touch the floor to complete 1 rep. You can increase the range of motion by placing weight plates underneath the front portion of your feet.

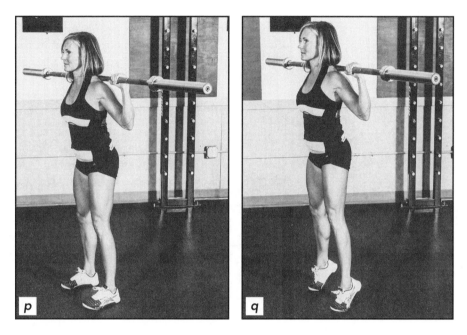

Wide-Grip Romanian Deadlift ▪ High Pull ▪ Front Squat ▪ Overhead Push Press ▪ Good Morning ▪ Reverse Lunge ▪ Shoulder Shrug ▪ Bent-Over Row

1 WIDE-GRIP ROMANIAN DEADLIFT

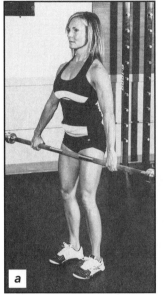
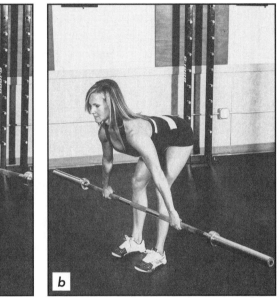

With your feet roughly hip-width apart, hold a barbell in front of your thighs with your arms straight, gripping the bar at a width about 5 inches outside shoulder-width apart (see figure a). Keeping your back straight, hinge at your hips and bend forward toward the floor, keeping your knees bent at roughly a 20-degree angle (see figure b). As you hinge forward, drive your hips backward and do not allow your back to round out. Once your torso is roughly parallel to the floor or the weight plates lightly tap the floor, drive your hips forward toward the barbell, reversing the motion to stand tall again and to complete 1 rep.

2 HIGH PULL

Slightly bend your knees and hinge forward at your hips with the barbell resting on your thighs (see figure c). Explode your body upward, pulling the bar toward the sky (see figure d), using your arms and legs simultaneously until your elbows reach shoulder height. Then lower the bar back to your thighs in a controlled fashion to reset and begin your next repetition.

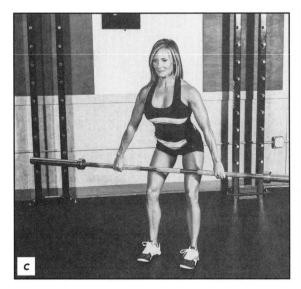
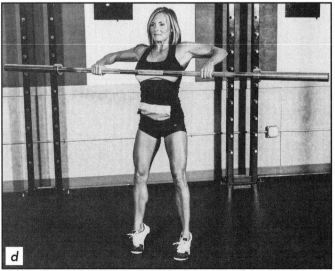

3 FRONT SQUAT

With the bar resting on the top of your chest and your elbows pointing straight out in front of you so they are parallel to the floor (see figure e), perform a squat, dropping as low as you possibly can while maintaining optimal control of your knee and spinal alignment (see figure f). Reverse the motion by standing up to begin the next repetition of this complex.

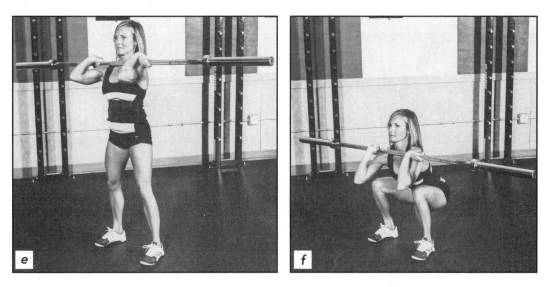

4 OVERHEAD PUSH PRESS

Stand with your feet shoulder-width apart and hold the barbell with your hands just outside shoulder-width apart (see figure g). Slightly bend your knees (see figure h) and then quickly reverse the motion, exploding into the bar and driving it overhead using both your arms and legs in a coordinated fashion (see figure i). Once the bar is completely overhead, slowly lower the barbell back down to complete 1 full repetition.

Note: After performing your last overhead push press, lower the barbell behind your head and place it across your shoulders to set up for the next exercise, good morning.

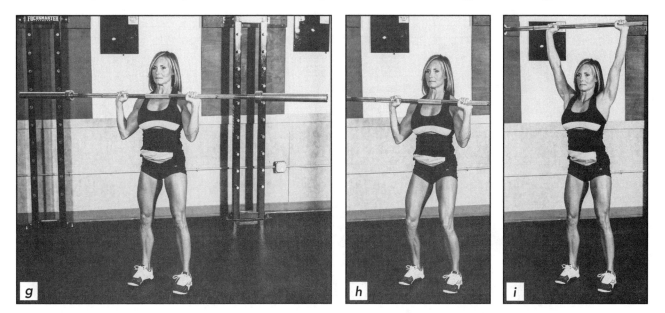

5 GOOD MORNING

Stand tall with your feet hip-width apart and place a barbell across your shoulders behind your head (see figure *j*). Keeping your back straight, hinge at your hips and bend forward toward the floor, keeping your knees bent at roughly a 15- to 20-degree angle (see figure *k*). As you hinge forward, drive your hips backward and do not allow your back to round out. Once your torso is roughly parallel to the floor, drive your hips forward toward the barbell, reversing the motion to stand tall again and complete 1 rep.

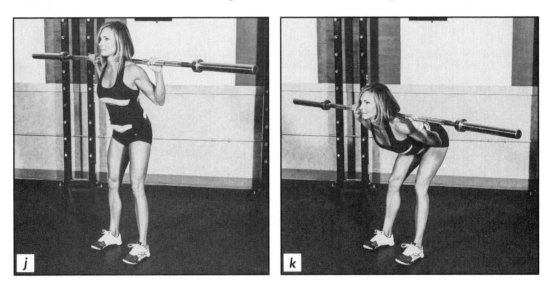

6 REVERSE LUNGE

Stand tall with your feet hip-width apart and a barbell across your shoulders behind your head (see figure *l*). Step backward with your right foot and drop your body so your knee lightly touches the floor (see figure *m*). Reverse the movement by coming out of the lunge and bringing your right foot forward so that you are back to your starting position. Perform the same movement on the opposite leg.

    Note: After performing your least reverse lunge repetition, drive the barbell of your shoulders using your arms and legs in a coordinated fashion. Bring the barbell in front of your body and lower it in front of your thighs to begin performing shoulder shrug.

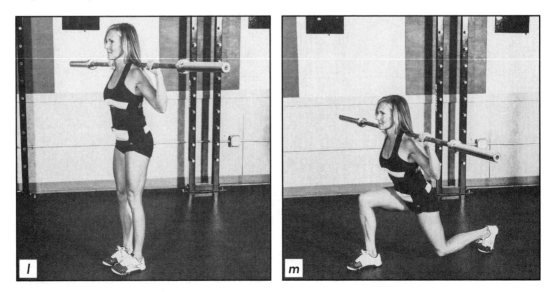

7 SHOULDER SHRUG

Stand tall with your feet hip-width apart, holding a barbell in front of your thighs with your hands just outside hip-width apart (see figure *n*). Shrug your shoulders up toward the sky as if to touch your shoulders to your ears (see figure *o*). Then lower the bar to the starting position to complete 1 rep. Be sure to keep your arms straight throughout the exercise.

Note: After finishing your shoulder shrugs, place the barbell on the floor and switch to an underhand grip to perform the next exercise, bent-over rows.

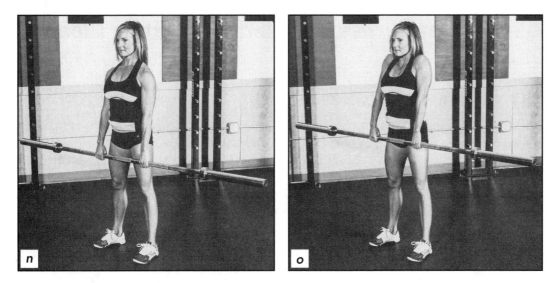

8 BENT-OVER ROW

Stand with your feet roughly hip-width apart. Hold the barbell using an underhand grip, keeping your hands just outside shoulder-width apart. Bend over at your hips, keeping your back straight so that your torso is parallel to the floor and your knees are bent 15 to 20 degrees (see figure *p*). Row the bar into the middle of your torso between your chest and your belly button (see figure *q*). Slowly lower the bar without allowing it to touch the ground to complete 1 rep. You can also perform bent-over rows by using an overhand grip, which many people find to be a less strong gripping option.

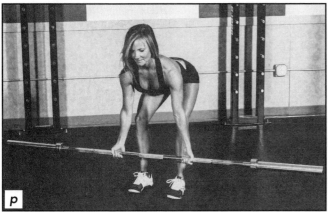
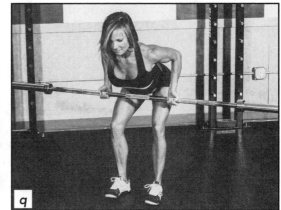

Angled Barbell Complexes

The following complexes involve placing one end of a barbell in a corner or inside a Sorinex Landmine device (www.sorinex.com) and holding the other end of the barbell. These angled barbell complexes are not only a great way to accelerate your metabolism and add some new metabolic strength training exercises to your routine to give you a challenge, but they're also sure to impress the know-it-alls at your gym.

Angled Reverse Lunge ▪ Angled Shoulder-to-Shoulder Press ▪ Angled Deadlift to Clean

1 ANGLED REVERSE LUNGE

With the barbell in front of you, stand tall with your feet hip-width apart. Hold onto the end of the barbell with both hands stacked one over the other and with the bar against the middle of your chest (see figure a). Step backward with your left foot and drop your body so your knee lightly touches the floor (see figure b). Reverse the movement by coming out of the lunge and bringing your right foot forward so that you are back to the starting position. Perform the same movement on the opposite leg.

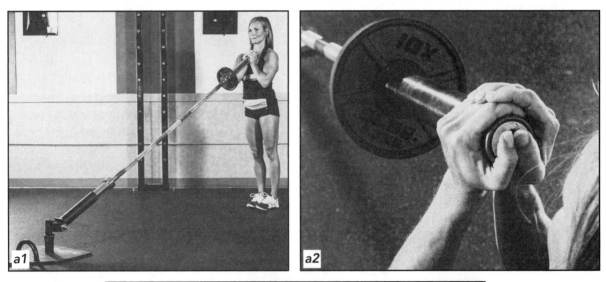

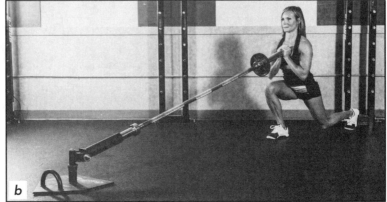

2 ANGLED SHOULDER-TO-SHOULDER PRESS

Stand tall with your feet parallel to one another and a little wider than shoulder-width apart. Hold onto the end of the barbell with both hands stacked one over the other and with the end of the barbell in front of your left shoulder (see figure c). Press the barbell out and away from you so that when your arms reach full extension, the barbell is directly in line with the center of your body (see figure d). Slowly reverse the motion and lower the barbell to your right shoulder (see figure e). Press it out and away again so that it ends up in the middle of your body. Make sure you do not allow your shoulders or hips to rotate throughout this exercise.

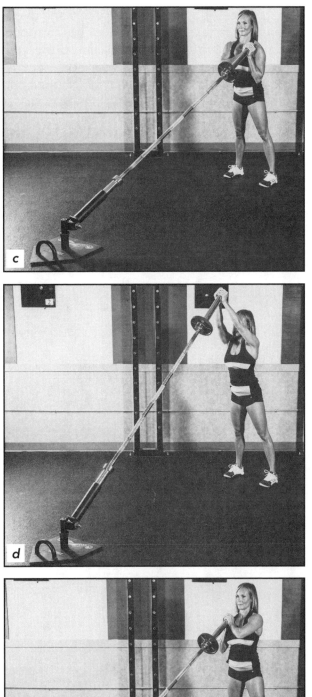

3 ANGLED DEADLIFT TO CLEAN

With your feet shoulder-width apart, stand over the weighted end of the barbell with the weight plates that are loaded onto the end of the barbell closest to the inside of your right foot (see figure f). Grasp the end of the barbell using a mixed grip, taking an overhand grip with your right hand and an underhand grip with your left hand. Lower your body into a deadlift position by bending your knees and hinging forward at your hips while keeping your back straight (see figure g). Stand up, lifting the bar off the floor while simultaneously exploding your hips forward into the bar and using your arms to pull the bar to your right shoulder so that the end of the barbell ends up in front of your chest and your elbows are underneath it (see figure h). Perform all reps on the same side before switching sides to repeat the exercise on the side of the body.

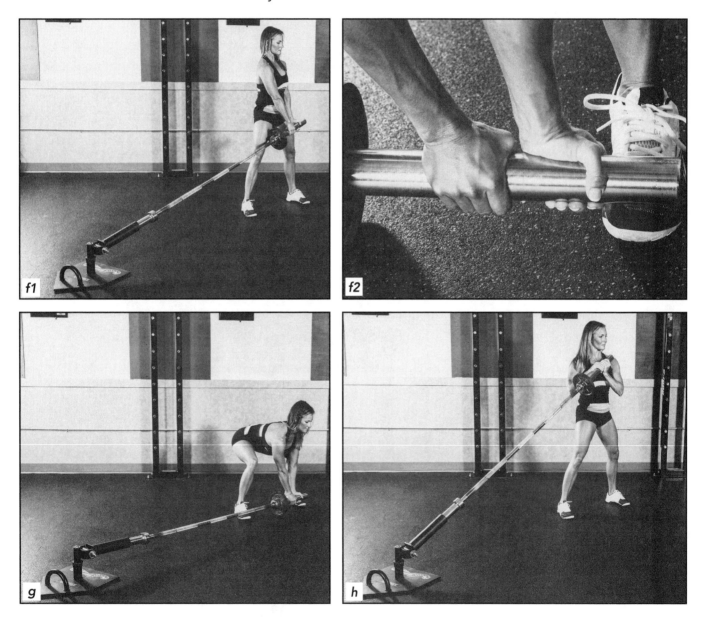

f1

f2

g

h

Angled Reverse Lunge to One-Arm Press ■
Angled Deadlift to Clean to Rotary Press ■
Angled One-Arm Row

1 ANGLED REVERSE LUNGE TO ONE-ARM PRESS

Stand tall facing the barbell with your feet hip-width apart. Hold the end of the barbell in your right hand with your elbow bent so that the barbell is at shoulder level (see figure a). Step backward with your right leg to perform a reverse lunge, allowing your right knee to gently touch the floor (see figure b). As you reverse the motion and begin to step forward out of the lunge, simultaneously press the bar out and away from you, keeping it in line with your right shoulder (see figure c). At the top of the exercise you should be in a parallel stance with your right arm fully extended. To repeat this exercise on the other side, switch the barbell to your left hand, bend your arm and slowly allow the barbell to lower toward your left shoulder as you simultaneously step your left leg back into the lunge. Perform all reps on the same side before switching sides.

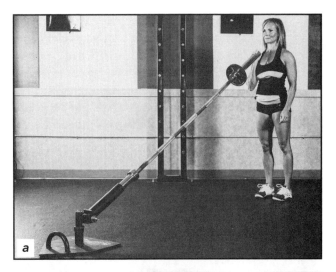

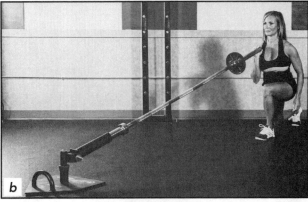

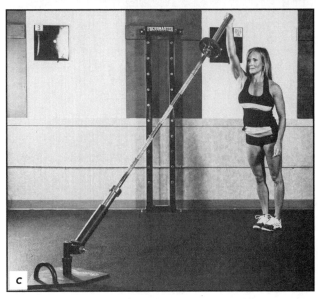

2 ANGLED DEADLIFT TO CLEAN TO ROTARY PRESS

With your feet slightly wider than shoulder-width apart, stand over the weighted end of the barbell with weight plates that are loaded onto the end of the barbell closest to the inside of your right foot and grasp the end of the barbell using a mixed grip, taking an overhand grip with your right hand and an underhand grip with your left hand (see figure d). Lower your body into a deadlift position by bending your knees and hinging forward at your hips while keeping your back straight (see figure e). Stand up, lifting the bar off the floor while simultaneously exploding your hips forward into the bar and using your arms to pull the bar to your left shoulder so that the end of the barbell ends up in front of your chest and your elbows are underneath it (see figure f). Then, with the bar at your chest, rotate your body (hips and torso) toward where the barbell is anchored (see figure g) as you push it away from you by extending both arms straight (see figure h). Slowly reverse the previous motions by first lowering the barbell to your chest and then to the floor in order to complete 1 repetition. Perform all reps on the same side before switching to the other side.

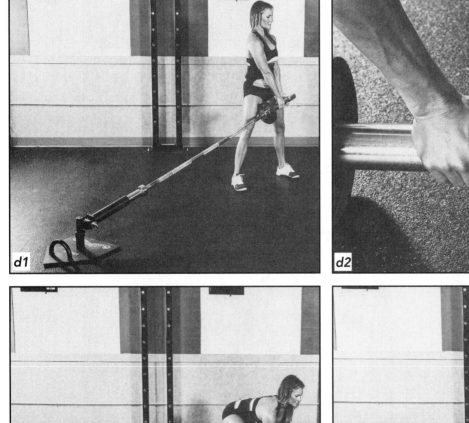

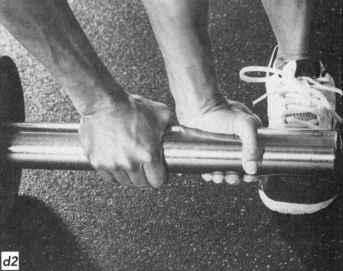

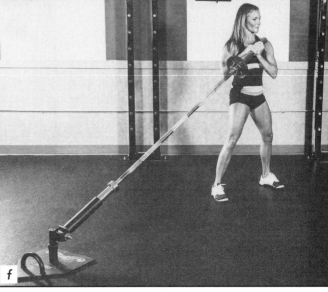

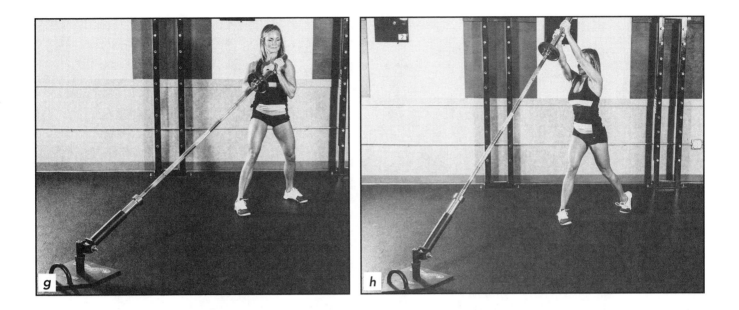

3 ANGLED ONE-ARM ROW

With your feet hip-width apart, stand parallel to the barbell so that the end of the barbell is in front of your right foot (or you can perform an angled row where you stand perpendicular to the bar). Bend your knees slightly, hinge forward at your hips while keeping your back straight, and grab the end of the barbell with your right hand (see figure *i*). Perform a one-arm row by pulling the barbell with your right hand into the right side of your body, keeping your elbow pointing toward the sky (see figure *j*). Once your elbow becomes parallel with your right shoulder, reverse the motion and slowly lower the end of the barbell until your elbow straightens. Perform all reps on the same side before switching sides.

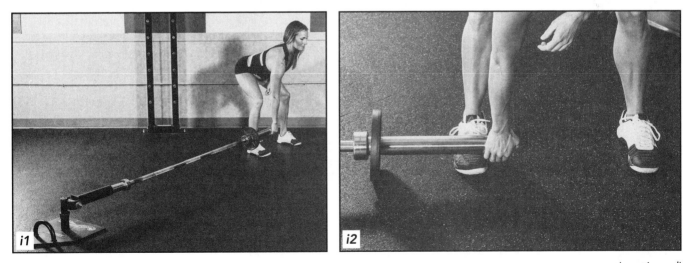

(continued)

(continued)

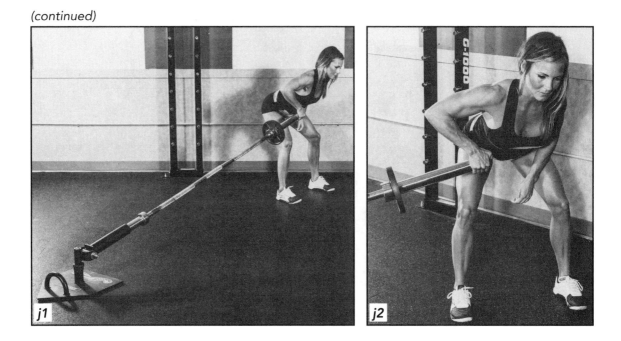

Dumbbell Complexes

Many of the following dumbbell complexes emphasize unilateral exercises, which, as discussed previously, automatically activate the core musculature in order to maintain your posture and body position to control the offset load. In addition, unilateral strength training exercises also ensure that both sides of the body get equal work. This is valuable because it's not uncommon for one side to be stronger than the other. With one-sided exercises, your weak side is forced to work and improve its strength relative to the other side.

Uppercut ▪ Squat to Romanian Deadlift ▪ Freestanding One-Arm Row

1 UPPERCUT

Stand tall with your feet roughly shoulder-width apart while holding a dumbbell in front of each shoulder (see figure *a*). Press one dumbbell into the air as you rotate to the opposite side (see figure *b*). Reverse the motion and press while rotating to the other side. To better allow your hips to rotate in this exercise, allow your heel to come off the ground as you turn.

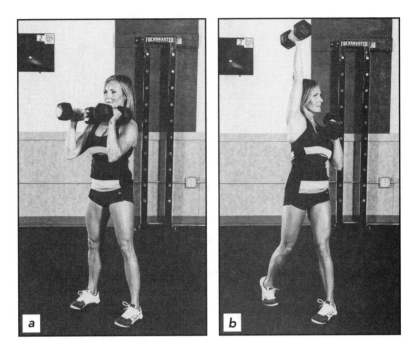

2 SQUAT TO ROMANIAN DEADLIFT

Stand tall with your feet hip-width apart and your toes pointed straight ahead. Hold a dumbbell in each hand at your sides by your hips (see figure *c*). Perform a squat by bending your knees and sitting back at your hips (see figure *d*). Go as low as you can possibly go without allowing your lower back to round out. As you squat, be sure that

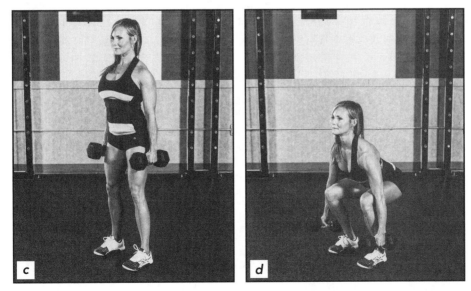

(continued)

(continued)

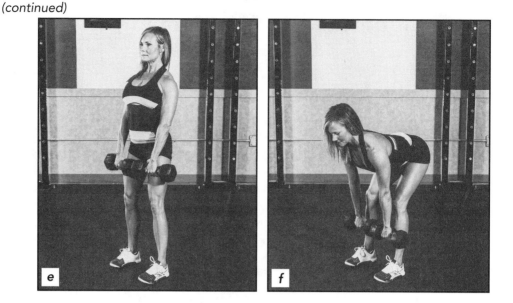

you do not allow your heels to come off the ground or your knees to come together toward the midline. Stand tall again and bring the dumbbells in front of your thighs (see figure *e*). Keep your back straight, hinge at your hips and bend forward toward the floor, keeping your knees bent at roughly a 15- to 20-angle (see figure *f*). As you hinge forward, drive your hips backward and do not allow your back to round out. Once your torso is roughly parallel to the floor, drive your hips forward toward the dumbbells, reversing the motion to stand tall again.

Note: After you finish all of your squat to Romanian deadlifts, place one dumbbell on the floor to set up to perform the next exercise, freestanding one-arm row.

3 FREESTANDING ONE-ARM ROW

Assume a split-stance position, with your right leg in front of your left leg with both knees slightly bent, and hold a dumbbell with your left hand. Hinge at your hips, keeping your back straight so that your torso becomes parallel with the floor (see figure *g*). Perform a row, pulling the dumbbell toward your body without rotating the shoulders or hips, making sure to pull your scapula toward your spine in a controlled manner as your arm moves into your body (see figure *h*). Be sure to maintain a stable spinal position, keeping your back straight throughout the exercise. Slowly lower the dumbbell toward the floor without letting it touch the floor. Repeat on the other side.

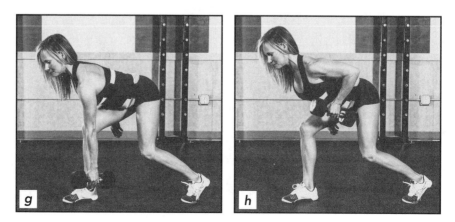

Bent-Over Row ▪ One-Leg Romanian Deadlift ▪
Front Squat ▪ Push-Up to Plank Row

1 BENT-OVER ROW

Stand with your feet roughly hip-width apart. Hold a dumbbell in each hand using a neutral grip so your palms are facing one another, keeping your hands just outside shoulder-width apart. Bend over at your hips, keeping your back straight so that your torso is parallel to the floor and your knees are bent 15 to 20 degrees (see figure a). Row the dumbbells into your sides at belly-button level (see figure b). Slowly lower the dumbbells until your arms are straight to complete 1 rep.

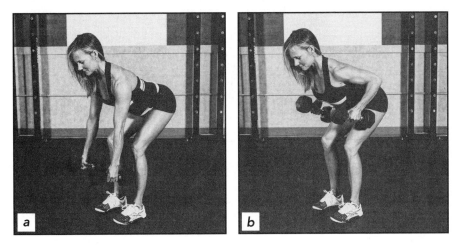

2 ONE-LEG ROMANIAN DEADLIFT

Stand on one leg, holding a dumbbell in each hand (see figure c). Keeping your back and both arms straight, hinge at your hip and bend forward toward the floor, keeping your weight-bearing knee bent at roughly a 15- to 20-degree angle (see figure d). As you hinge, allow your non-weight-bearing leg to elevate so it remains in a straight line with your torso while also not allowing your lower back to round out. At the bottom position (when your torso is roughly parallel to the ground), be sure to keep your hips flat and do not allow them to rotate. Once your torso and non-weight-bearing leg are roughly parallel to the floor, reverse the motion by driving your hips forward to stand tall again and complete 1 rep. Switch your stance leg on each rep.

Note: After performing your last one-leg Romanian deadlift repetition, use your legs to help you lift the dumb-bells in front of your shoulders to set up for the front squat.

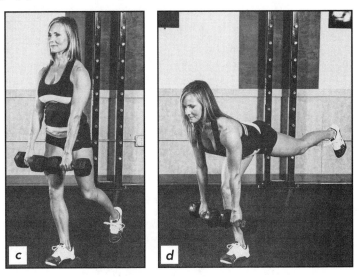

③ FRONT SQUAT

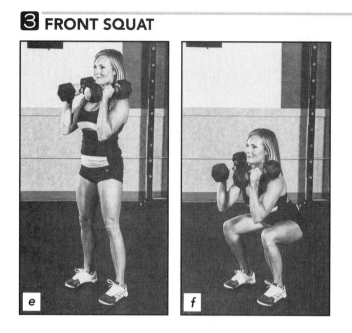

Stand tall with your feet shoulder-width apart. Hold a dumbbell in each hand at your shoulders with your elbows directly underneath the handles of the dumbbells (see figure *e*). Squat as low as you can by bending your knees and sitting your hips back without allowing your heels to rise off the floor or allowing your lower back to round out (see figure *f*). Reverse the motion and return to the tall standing position.

④ PUSH-UP TO PLANK ROW

Assume a plank push-up position with one hand on the handle of each dumbbell, directly under your shoulders (see figure *g*). Perform a push-up by lowering your body to the floor while keeping your elbows directly above your wrists the entire time (see figure *h*). Once your ribs come in contact with the dumbbells, reverse the motion by pushing your body up (see figure *i*). Do not allow your head or hips to sag toward the floor at any time. From the top of push-up position, row the left dumbbell up into your body until it touches your ribs (see figure *j*). Slowly lower the dumbbell back to the floor and row the right dumbbell in the same manner. While rowing the dumbbells, be sure your torso remains as stable as possible; do not allow your hips to rotate at any time.

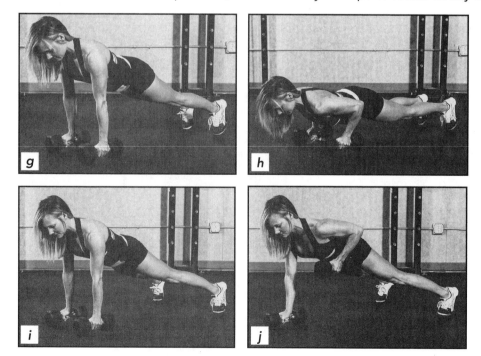

Freestanding One-Arm Row ▪ Suitcase Squat ▪ One-Arm Overhead Push Press

In this complex, all of the exercises are performed on the same side before switching sides. Following are the exercises for this complex.

1 FREESTANDING ONE-ARM ROW

Assume a split-stance position, with your right leg in front of your left leg with both knees slightly bent, and hold a dumbbell with your left hand. Hinge at your hips, keeping your back straight so that your torso becomes parallel with the floor (see figure a). Perform a row, pulling the dumbbell toward your body without rotating the shoulders or hips, making sure to pull your scapula toward your spine in a controlled manner as your arm moves into your body (see figure b). Be sure to maintain a stable spinal position, keeping your back straight throughout the exercise. Slowly lower the dumbbell toward the floor without letting it touch the floor. Repeat on the other side.

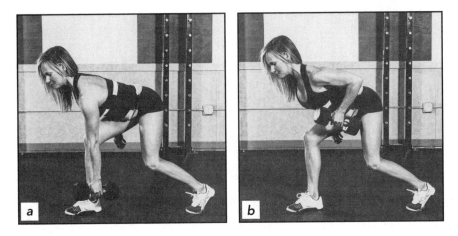

2 SUITCASE SQUAT

Stand tall with your feet hip-width apart and your toes pointed straight ahead. Hold one dumbbell at your side by your hip (see figure c). Perform a squat by bending your knees and sitting back at your hips (see figure d). Go as low as you can possibly go without allowing your lower back to round out. As you squat, do not allow your heels to come off the ground or your knees to come together toward the midline. Your knees should track in the same direction as your toes.

Note: After performing your last suitcase squat repetition, use your free hand to help you lift the dumbbell in front of your shoulder to set up for the one-arm overhead push press.

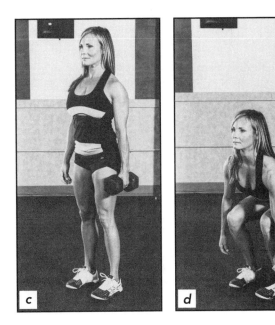

❸ ONE-ARM OVERHEAD PUSH PRESS

Stand tall with your feet roughly shoulder-width apart while holding a dumbbell in your left hand at shoulder level with your left elbow directly below the handle of the dumbbell (see figure e). Slightly bend your knees (see figure f), and use your legs simultaneously with your left arm to explode upward and press the dumbbell overhead (see figure g). Slowly lower the dumbbell to your shoulder to complete 1 rep.

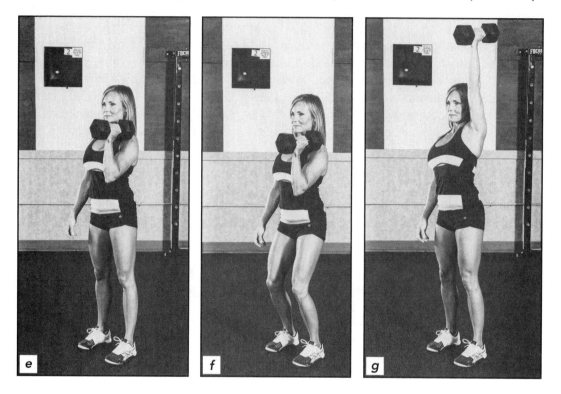

One-Arm Uppercut ▪ Reverse Lunge With Dumbbell at Shoulder ▪ One-Arm Swing ▪ One-Leg One-Arm Romanian Deadlift

This complex requires you to perform all exercises with the dumbbell on the same side before switching sides. Following are the exercises for this complex.

1 ONE-ARM UPPERCUT

Stand tall with your feet roughly shoulder-width apart while holding a dumbbell in front of one shoulder (see figure a). Press the dumbbell into the air as you rotate to the side opposite the dumbbell (see figure b). To better allow your hips to rotate in this exercise, allow your right heel to come off the ground as you turn.

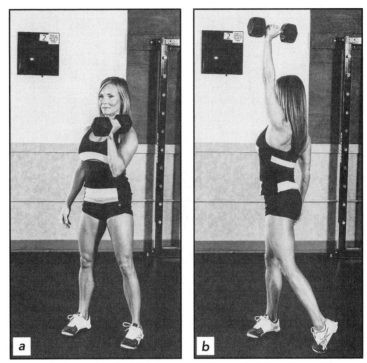

2 REVERSE LUNGE WITH DUMBBELL AT SHOULDER

Stand with your feet hip-width apart and hold a dumbbell at your left shoulder (see figure c). Step backward with your left foot and drop your body so your knee lightly touches the floor (see figure d). Reverse the movement by coming out of the lunge and bringing your left foot forward so that you are back to your starting position.

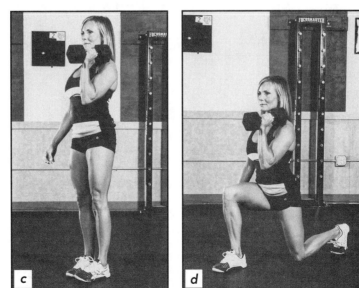

3 ONE-ARM SWING

With your feet roughly hip-width apart, hold a dumbbell in one hand. Keeping your back and arm straight, drive the dumbbell between your legs as if hiking a football and hinge forward at your hips, keeping your knees bent at roughly a 15- to 20-degree angle (see figure e). Once your forearm comes into contact with your same-side thigh, explosively reverse the motion by simultaneously driving your hips forward and swinging the dumbbell upward to eye level to complete 1 rep (see figure f).

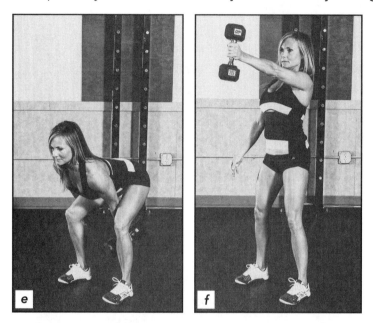

As you hinge forward, be sure that you drive your hips backward and do not allow your back to round out. Also, allowing your forearm to touch the inside of your same-side thigh at the bottom of each swing ensures that you're doing the exercise properly by emphasizing a powerful involvement of your lower-body leg and hip musculature instead of just lifting the dumbbell with your arm.

4 ONE-LEG ONE-ARM ROMANIAN DEADLIFT

Stand on your right leg and hold a dumbbell in your left hand (see figure g). Keeping your back and left arm straight, hinge at your hip and bend forward toward the floor, keeping your weight-bearing knee bent at roughly a 15- to 20-degree angle (see figure h). As you hinge, allow your non-weight-bearing leg to elevate upward so it remains in a straight line with your torso, and do not allow your lower back to round out. At the bottom position (when your torso is roughly parallel to the ground), be sure to keep your hips flat and do not allow them to rotate. Once your torso and non-weight-bearing leg are roughly parallel to the floor, reverse the motion by driving your hips forward to stand tall again, completing 1 rep.

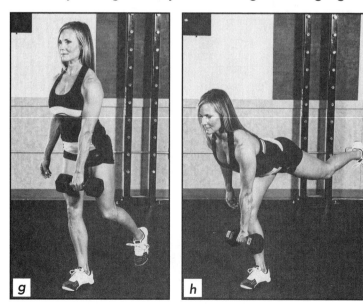

Squat Jump ▪ Push-Up to Plank Row ▪ Two-Arm Swing ▪ Uppercut ▪ Bent-Over Row

1 SQUAT JUMP

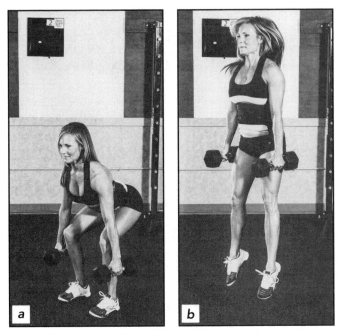

With your feet roughly shoulder-width apart, stand tall holding one dumbbell in each hand outside your hips and squat so that your thighs are parallel or slightly below parallel with the floor, making sure you do not allow your lower back to round out (see figure a). Explode up by extending your legs and jumping into the air (see figure b). Land as lightly and as quietly as possible into a squat position. Make sure that each time you squat down your knees remain in the same line as your toes; your knees should not come toward one another at any time.

2 PUSH-UP TO PLANK ROW

Assume a plank push-up position with one hand on the handle of each dumbbell, directly under your shoulders (see figure c). Perform a push-up by lowering your body to the floor while keeping your elbows directly above your wrists the entire time (see figure d). Once your ribs come in contact with the dumbbells, reverse the motion by pushing your body up (see figure e). Do not allow your head or hips to sag toward the floor at any time. From the top of push-up position, row the left dumbbell up into your body until it touches your ribs (see figure f). Slowly lower the dumbbell back to the floor and row the right dumbbell in the same manner. While rowing the dumbbells, be sure your torso remains as stable as possible; do not allow your hips to rotate at any time.

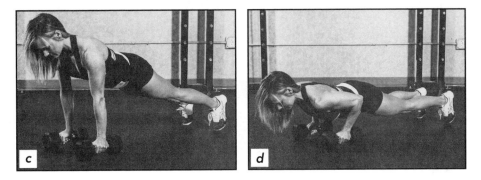

(continued)

(continued)

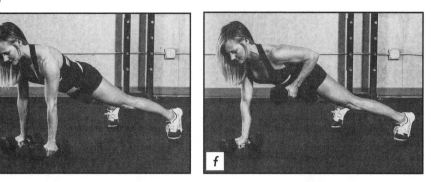

❸ TWO-ARM SWING

With your feet roughly hip-width apart, hold a dumbbell in each hand. Keeping your back and arms straight, drive the dumbbells between your legs as if hiking a football and hinge forward at your hips, keeping your knees bent at roughly a 15- to 20-degree angle (see figure g). Once your forearms come into contact with your thighs, explosively reverse the motion by simultaneously driving your hips forward and swinging the dumbbells upward to eye level to complete 1 rep (see figure h).

As you hinge forward, be sure that you drive your hips backward and do not allow your back to round out. Also, allow your forearms to touch the insides of your thighs at the bottom of each swing. Use your hips to powerfully drive your arms forward off your thighs to swing the dumbbells up on each rep. This ensures that you're doing the exercise properly by emphasizing a powerful involvement of your lower-body leg and hip musculature instead of just lifting the dumbbell with your arms. On your last rep, swing the dumbbells up to your shoulders to set up for the next exercise.

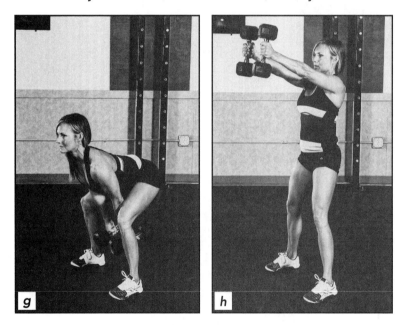

4 UPPERCUT

Stand tall with your feet roughly shoulder-width apart while holding a dumbbell in front of each shoulder (see figure *i*). Press one dumbbell into the air as you rotate to the opposite side (see figure *j*). Reverse the motion and repeat while rotating to the other side. To better allow your hips to rotate in this exercise, allow your heel to come off the ground as you turn.

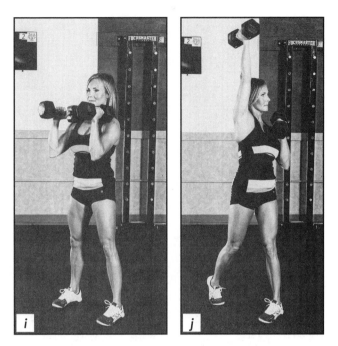

5 BENT-OVER ROW

Stand with your feet roughly hip-width apart. Hold a dumbbell in each hand using a neutral grip so your palms are facing one another, keeping your hands just outside shoulder-width apart. Bend over at your hips, keeping your back straight so that your torso is parallel to the floor and your knees are bent 15 to 20 degrees (see figure *k*). Row the dumbbells into your sides at belly-button level (see figure *l*). Slowly lower the dumbbells until your arms are straight to complete 1 rep.

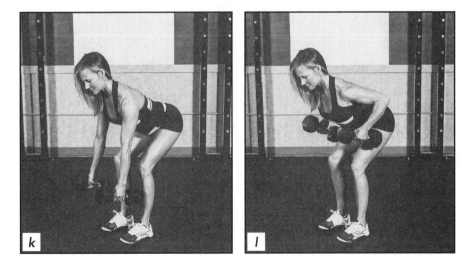

Front Squat ▪ Uppercut ▪ Two-Arm Swing ▪ Push-Up to Plank Row ▪ Turkish Get-Up

1 FRONT SQUAT

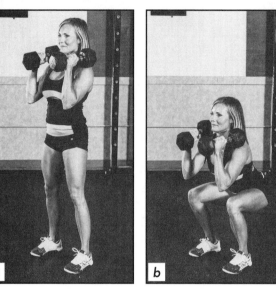

Stand tall with your feet shoulder-width apart. Hold a dumbbell in each hand at your shoulders with your elbows directly underneath the handles of the dumbbells (see figure a). Squat as low as you can by bending your knees and sitting your hips back without allowing your heels to rise off the floor or allowing your lower back to round out (see figure b). Reverse the motion and return to the tall standing position.

2 UPPERCUT

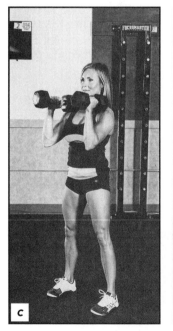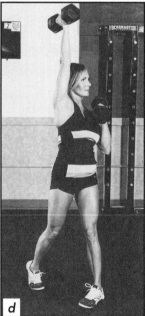

Stand tall with your feet roughly shoulder-width apart while holding a dumbbell in front of each shoulder (see figure c). Press one dumbbell into the air as you rotate to the opposite side (see figure d). Reverse the motion and repeat while rotating to the other side. To better allow your hips to rotate in this exercise, allow your heel to come off the ground as you turn.

3 TWO-ARM SWING

With your feet roughly hip-width apart, hold a dumb-bell in each hand. Keeping your back and arms straight, drive the dumbbells between your legs as if hiking a football and hinge forward at your hips, keeping your knees bent at roughly a 15- to 20-degree angle (see figure e). Once your forearms come into contact with your thighs, explosively reverse the motion by simultaneously driving your hips forward and swinging the dumbbells upward to eye level to complete 1 rep (see figure f).

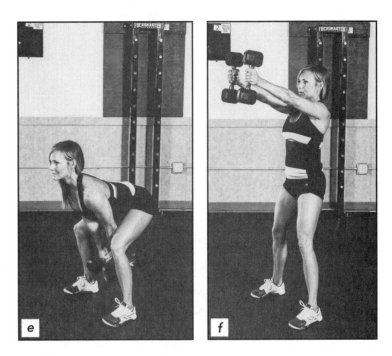

As you hinge forward, be sure that you drive your hips backward and do not allow your back to round out. Also, allow your forearms to touch the insides of your thighs at the bottom of each swing. Use your hips to powerfully drive your arms forward off your thighs to swing the dumbbells up on each rep. This ensures that you're doing the exercise properly by emphasizing a powerful involvement of your lower-body leg and hip musculature instead of just lifting the dumbbell with your arms.

4 PUSH-UP TO PLANK ROW

Assume a plank push-up position with one hand on the handle of each dumbbell, directly under your shoulders (see figure g). Perform a push-up by lowering your body to the floor while keeping your elbows directly above your wrists the entire time (see figure h). Once your ribs come in contact with the dumbbells, reverse the motion by pushing your body up (see figure i). Do not allow your head or hips to sag toward the floor at any time. From the top of push-up position, row the left dumbbell up into your body until it touches your ribs (see figure j). Slowly lower the dumbbell back to the floor and row the right dumbbell in the same manner. While rowing the dumbbells, be sure your torso remains as stable as possible; do not allow your hips to rotate at any time.

Note: After you've completed all the reps of the push-up to plank row, roll one dumbbell away from you and roll to your back (holding the other dumbbell in one hand) to set up for the next exercise, Turkish get-up.

(continued)

(continued)

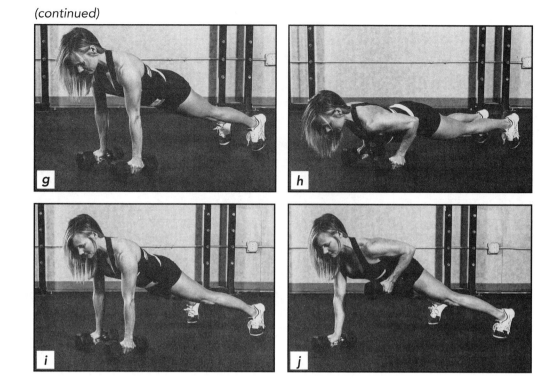

5️⃣ TURKISH GET-UP

Although the Turkish get-up has a single name, it is truly a combination of several exercises that can be done while holding a dumbbell (or kettlebell). If you've never tried the Turkish get-up, get ready for an exercise that's unlike any other.

Lie supine on the floor, holding a dumbbell (or kettlebell) in your left hand. Reach your arm toward the sky directly above your shoulder and bend your left knee (see figure *k*). Roll to your right elbow, keeping your left arm stable (see figure *l*). Then extend your right elbow to sit up (see figure *m*). Raise your hips into the air (see figure *n*) and slide your right leg underneath your body (see figure *o*), placing your right knee on the floor while continuing to keep your left arm straight and stable (see figure *p*). Then raise your torso so that it's perpendicular to the floor (see figure *q*).

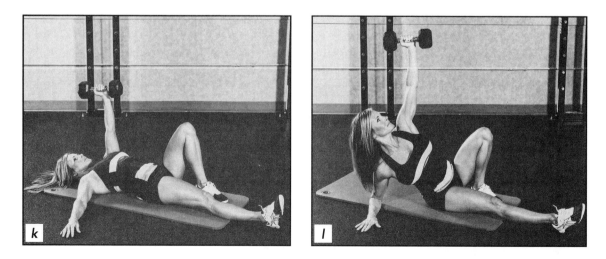

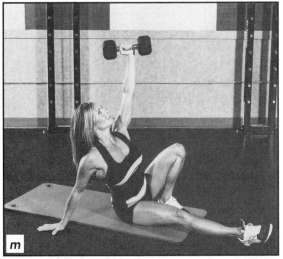

m

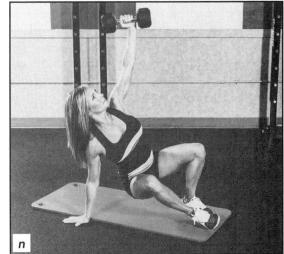

n

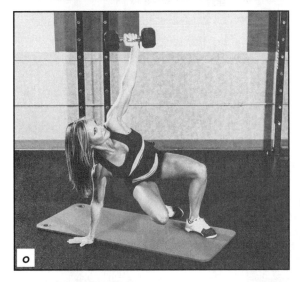

o

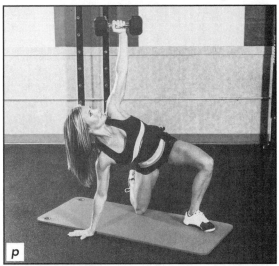

p

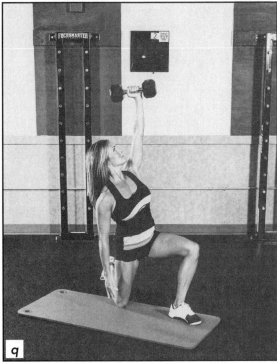

q

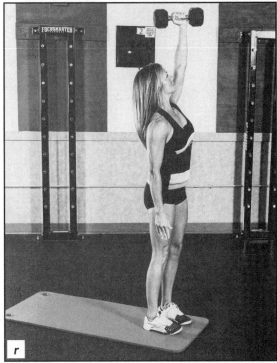

r

(continued)

(continued)
Finally, stand up out of the half-kneeling position (see figure *r*). Then slowly reverse each motion step by step until you're in the starting position in order to complete 1 rep. Repeat on the other side. Note that you can switch hands after each rep or switch sides every two, three, or four reps and so on—whatever you feel is needed to maintain optimal intensity and control when performing the exercise.

Uppercut ▪ Reverse Lunge ▪ High Pull ▪ One-Leg Romanian Deadlift

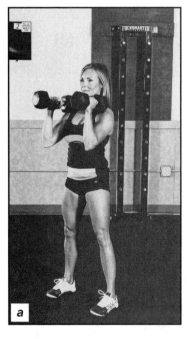
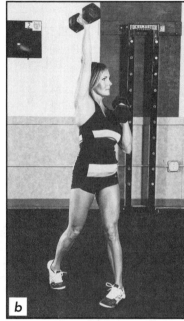

1 UPPERCUT

Stand tall with your feet roughly shoulder-width apart while holding a dumbbell in front of each shoulder (see figure *a*). Press one dumbbell into the air as you rotate to the opposite side (see figure *b*). Reverse the motion and press while rotating to the other side. To better allow your hips to rotate in this exercise, allow your heel to come off the ground as you turn.

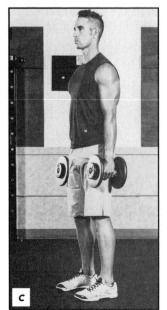
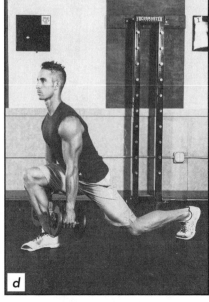

2 REVERSE LUNGE

Stand with your feet hip-width apart and hold a dumbbell at your sides (see figure *c*). Step backward with your left foot and drop your body so your knee lightly touches the floor (see figure *d*). Reverse the movement by coming out of the lunge and bringing your left foot forward so that you are back to your starting position. Alternate legs on each repetition.

3 HIGH PULL

Stand with your feet hip-width apart and hold a dumbbell in each hand. Slightly hinge at your hips and slightly bend your knees (see figure e). Explosively drive your hips and knee straight while simultaneously pulling the dumbbells up, keeping your elbows pointing upward (see figure f). Once the dumbbells reach chest level, lower them to the starting position.

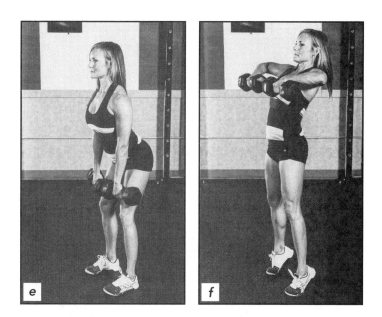

4 ONE-LEG ROMANIAN DEADLIFT

Stand on your right leg, holding a dumbbell in each hand (see figure g). Keeping your back and both arms straight, hinge at your hip and bend forward toward the floor, keeping your right knee bent at roughly a 15- to 20-degree angle (see figure h).

As you hinge, allow your non-weight-bearing leg to elevate so it remains in a straight line with your torso while also not allowing your lower back to round out. At the bottom position (when your torso is roughly parallel to the ground), be sure to keep your hips flat and do not allow them to rotate. Once your torso and non-weight-bearing leg are roughly parallel to the floor, reverse the motion by driving your hips forward to stand tall again and complete 1 rep. Repeat on the other leg.

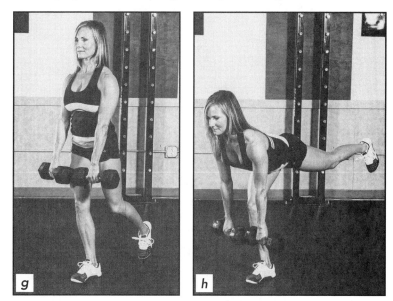

Kettlebell Complexes

The kettlebell is a very old exercise tool that has seen a resurgence in modern-day fitness training, and for good reason—it's a versatile tool that allows for unique exercise applications that nicely complement other modalities such as barbells, dumbbells, resistance bands, body-weight training, and so on. The beauty of the kettlebell design is that it allows for smooth transitions from one exercise to the next, as you'll see in the following complexes. It is recommended that you develop the ability to perform the fundamental kettlebell exercises, especially movements such as the swing clean, because they require a bit of practice to perform safely and effectively.

Two-Arm Swing ▪ Two-Arm Swing Clean ▪ Front Squat ▪ Two-Arm Overhead Push Press

1 TWO-ARM SWING

With your feet hip-width apart, hold a kettlebell in each hand. Keeping your back and arms straight, drive the kettlebells between your legs as if hiking a football and hinge forward at your hips, keeping your knees bent at roughly a 15- to 20-degree angle (see figure a). Once your forearms come into contact with your thighs, explosively reverse the motion by simultaneously driving your hips forward (see figure b) and swinging the kettlebells upward to eye level to complete 1 rep.

As you hinge forward, be sure that you drive your hips backward and do not allow your back to round out. Also, allow your forearms to touch the insides of your thighs at the bottom of each swing. Use your hips to powerfully drive your arms forward off your thighs to swing the kettlebells back up on each rep. This ensures that you're doing the exercise properly by emphasizing a powerful involvement of your lower-body and hip musculature instead of just lifting the kettlebells with your arms.

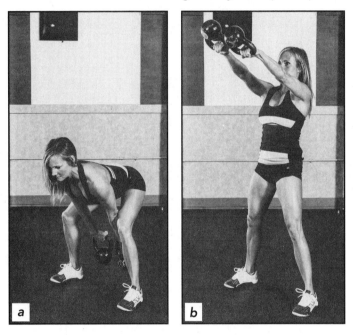

2 TWO-ARM SWING CLEAN

Stand with your feet wider than shoulder-width apart and hold a kettlebell in each hand. Slightly bend your knees and hinge at your hips to allow the kettlebells to swing between your legs (see figure c). Quickly reverse this motion by driving your hips forward and moving your arms upward (see figure d). As the kettlebells move toward the sky, quickly flip your elbows underneath them and soften your body to accept the kettlebells moving into your body, creating as much of a cushion as you can (see figures e and f). In other words, as the kettlebells come up to your chest, imagine that they're eggs that you do not want to break, absorbing them as gently as possible.

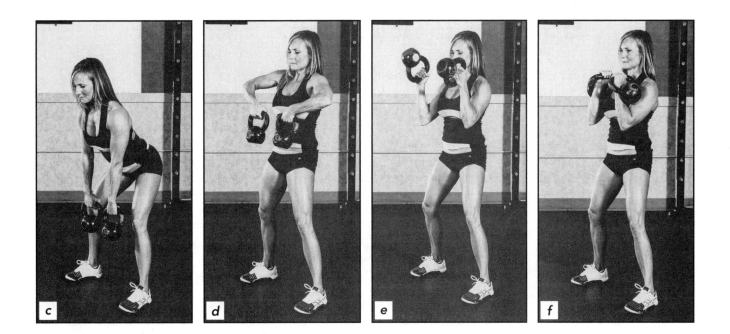

c d e f

❸ FRONT SQUAT

With your feet slightly wider than shoulder-width apart and toes turned out 10 to 15 degrees, hold the kettlebells in front of you, resting them on the top of your chest and forearms (see figure g). Your hands should be closer to the center of your chest and your elbows should be flared out to the sides of your body, pointing down like a triangle. Be sure to stay tall and lift your chest to create a rack for the kettlebells instead of trying to hold them up using only your arms. Bend at your knees and hips and lower

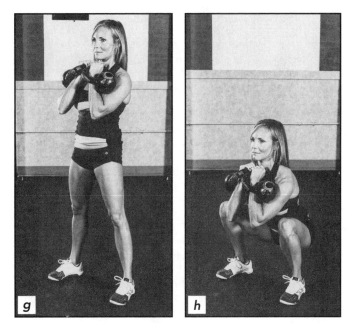

g h

your body toward the floor as low as you can possibly go (see figure h). As you drop into the squat, be sure to keep your elbows lifted high toward the sky. Your heels should not to lift off the ground and your lower back should not lose its arch. Also, be sure to keep your knees wide and tracking in the same direction as your toes and do not allow your knees to drop in toward the midline of your body. Once you've gone as deep as you can control in the squat, reverse the motion by standing up.

4 TWO-ARM OVERHEAD PUSH PRESS

Stand with your feet shoulder-width apart, holding the kettlebells with your hands just outside shoulder-width apart with the kettlebells resting on the top of your chest and forearms (see figure *i*). Your hands should be closer to the center of your chest and your elbows should be flared out to the sides of your body, pointing downward like a triangle. Slightly bend your knees (see figure *j*) and then quickly reverse the motion, exploding into the kettlebells by pressing them overhead using both your arms and legs in a coordinated fashion (see figure *k*). Once the kettlebells are completely overhead, slowly reverse the motion by lowering them to the starting position.

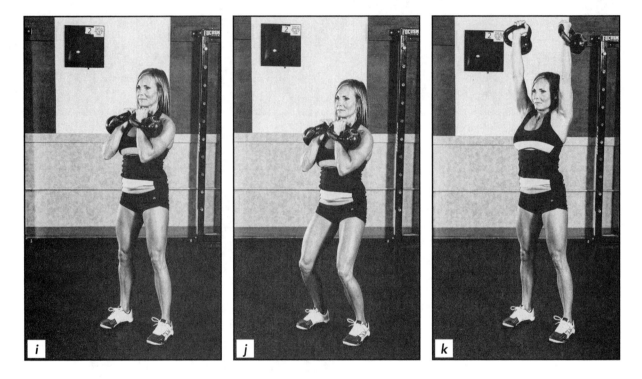

Two-Arm Overhead Push Press ▪
Reverse Lunge With Kettlebells at Shoulder ▪
Two-Arm Swing ▪ Bent-Over Row

1 TWO-ARM OVERHEAD PUSH PRESS

Stand with your feet shoulder-width apart, holding the kettlebells with your hands just outside shoulder-width apart with the kettlebells resting on the top of your chest and forearms (see figure *a*). Your hands should be closer to the center of your chest and your elbows should be flared out to the sides of your body, pointing downward like a triangle. Slightly bend your knees (see figure *b*) and then quickly reverse the motion, exploding into the kettlebells by pressing them overhead using both your arms and legs in a coordinated fashion (see figure *c*). Once the kettlebells are completely overhead, slowly reverse the motion by lowering them to the starting position.

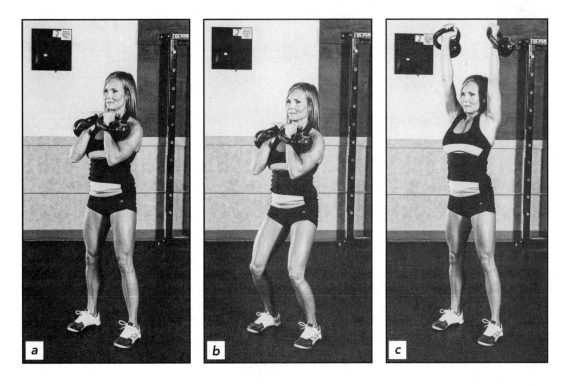

2 REVERSE LUNGE WITH KETTLEBELLS AT SHOULDER

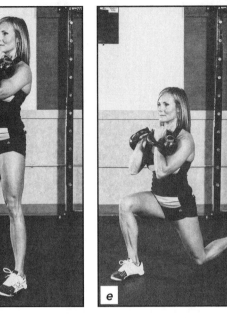

Stand with your feet hip-width apart and hold two kettlebells in front of you, resting them on the top of your chest and forearms (see figure *d*). Your hands should be closer to the center of your chest and your elbows should be pointing downward like a triangle. Step backward with your left foot and drop your body so your knee lightly touches the floor (see figure *e*). Reverse the movement by coming out of the lunge and bringing your left foot forward so that you are back to your starting position. Switch legs and repeat.

3 TWO-ARM SWING

With your feet hip-width apart, hold a kettlebell in each hand. Keeping your back and arms straight, drive the kettlebells between your legs as if hiking a football and hinge forward at your hips, keeping your knees bent at roughly a 15- to 20-degree angle (see figure *f*). Once your forearms come into contact with your thighs, explosively reverse the motion by simultaneously driving your hips forward (see figure *g*) and swinging the kettlebells upward to eye level to complete 1 rep.

As you hinge forward, be sure that you drive your hips backward and do not allow your back to round out. Also, allow your forearms to touch the insides of your thighs at the bottom of each swing. Use your hips to powerfully drive your arms forward off your thighs to swing the kettlebells back up on each rep. This ensures that you're doing the exercise properly by emphasizing a powerful involvement of your lower-body and hip musculature instead of just lifting the kettlebells with your arms.

4 BENT-OVER ROW

Stand with your feet roughly hip-width apart and hold a kettlebell in each hand just outside shoulder-width apart using a neutral grip so your palms are facing one another. Bend over at your hips, keeping your back straight so that your torso is parallel to the floor and your knees are bent 15 to 20 degrees (see figure *h*). Row the kettlebells into your sides at belly-button level (see figure *i*). Slowly lower the kettlebells until your arms are straight to complete 1 rep.

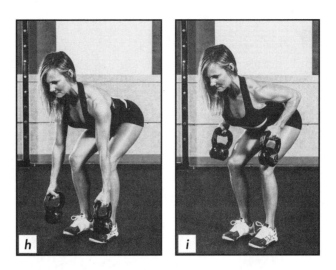

Weight-Plate Complex

The following complex requires you to hold each end of a 25-, 35-, or 45-pound Olympic-style weight plate, which is the traditional style of weight plate found most gyms. This complex is unique because it involves all total-body movements that are different from those featured previously. The following complex is dynamic and requires good amount of coordination and athleticism.

Diagonal Chop ▪ Middle Chop ▪ Lateral Lunge

1 DIAGONAL CHOP

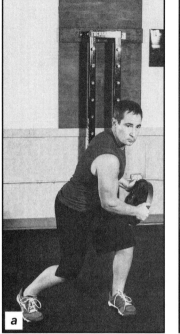

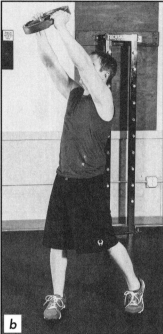

Squat down and rotate your hips and torso, holding the plate outside your left knee (see figure *a*). Stand up as you rotate to your right side and drive the plate across your body, finishing with it above your head (see figure *b*). This exercise should be performed in a smooth and rhythmic fashion, coordinating your upper body and lower body on the lifting and lowering phase of each repetition. Perform all reps in the same direction, then repeat the exercise on the other side.

2 MIDDLE CHOP

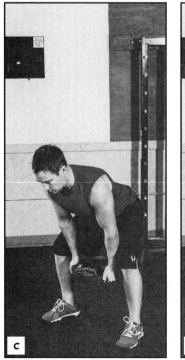

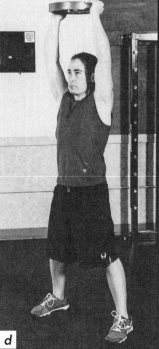

This exercise is performed virtually the same as the swing, with the exception that you finish with the plate overhead instead of at eye level. Squat down, holding the plate between your legs (see figure *c*). Stand up as you drive the plate up, finishing with it above your head (see figure *d*). This exercise should be performed in a smooth and rhythmic fashion, coordinating your upper body and lower body on the lifting and lowering phase of each repetition.

3 LATERAL LUNGE

Stand tall and hold a weight-plate at your chest with your feet hip-width apart (see figure e). Step about 3 to 4 feet to your left, squatting as low as you can go while maintaining good control, keeping your right leg straight and both feet flat on the floor (see figure f). Reverse the motion, stepping back so that your feet are together. Repeat by stepping out with your right leg.

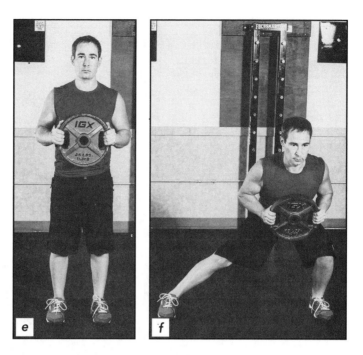

Hybrid Locomotion Complexes

In addition to the complexes covered previously, which are performed in one place, there are also complexes that involve locomotion, where you alternate loaded exercises (in place) with resisted locomotive exercise (moving up and down a room). There are two locomotive complexes: the farmer's walk and the plate push.

Farmer's Walk Complexes

A farmer's walk or farmer's carry complex is a series of dumbbell exercises interspersed between several sets of dumbbell carries. These complexes are performed back to back (circuit style) without rest until all exercises within a given complex have been completed.

There are two farmer's walk complexes—a bilateral version and a unilateral version. They both require two sets of dumbbells. You'll use a heavier set for the farmer's carry portions of each complex and a lighter set for the other exercises in the complex. The lighter set should be roughly 50 to 65 percent of the weight you used for the heavier pair. For example, if your heavier set is 80 pounds, then your lighter set should be around 45 pounds.

To set up this complex, place two cones 20 to 40 yards apart. Place both pairs of dumbbells at one end. During the farmer's carry in these complexes, the dumbbells are carried back and forth (20-25 yd.) between the two cones, so if you don't have much free space in your weight room, just bring some dumbbells into the group fitness room at your gym or go outside if the weather is okay.

The steps of the following complexes represent one set. For the bilateral version, perform 3 to 5 rounds with 2 to 3 minutes of rest between rounds. For the unilateral version, perform 2 to 3 rounds on each side (4-6 total sets) with 1 to 2 minutes of rest between sides. Regardless of whether you're performing a unilateral or bilateral complex, take long strides and move as fast as you can without losing control of the weight.

Bilateral Farmer's Walk Complex

1 FARMER'S WALK

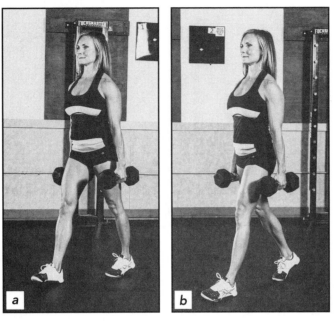

Stand next to one cone and hold two heavy dumbbells on each side of your body, with palms facing the body, either by your hips or at your shoulders (see figure *a* for an example at the hips). Walk to the opposite cone and return to your starting point, keeping the dumbbells in this position while maintaining a strong upright posture (see figure *b*).

2 BENT-OVER ROW

Stand next to one cone with your feet roughly hip-width apart. Hold a lighter dumbbell in each hand using a neutral grip so your palms are facing one another, keeping your hands just outside shoulder-width apart. Bend over at your hips, keeping your back straight so that your torso is parallel to the floor and your knees are bent 15 to 20 degrees (see figure *c*). Row the dumbbells into your sides at belly-button level (see figure *d*). Slowly lower the dumbbells until your arms are straight to complete 1 rep. Perform 6 to 8 reps total.

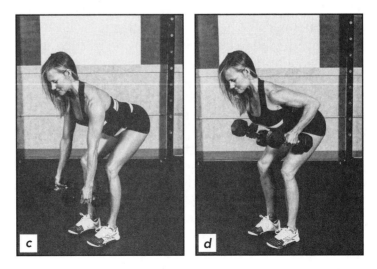

3 FARMER'S WALK

As described previously, stand next to one cone and hold two heavy dumbbells on each side of your body, with palms facing the body, either by your hips or at your shoulders. Walk to the opposite cone and return to your starting point, keeping the dumbbells in this position while maintaining a strong, upright posture.

4 OVERHEAD PRESS

Stand next to one cone with your feet roughly shoulder-width apart and hold the lighter dumbbells in each hand at shoulder level (see figure e). Press the dumbbells toward the sky, keeping your torso as stable as possible (see figure f). Slowly lower the dumbbells back to your shoulders to complete 1 rep. Perform 6 to 8 reps total.

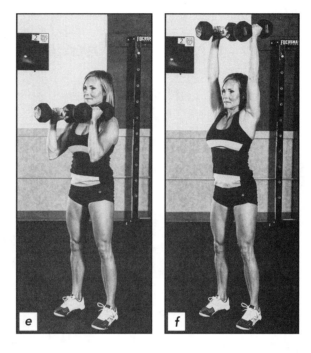

5 FARMER'S WALK

As described previously, stand next to one cone and hold two heavy dumbbells on each side of your body, with palms facing the body, either by your hips or at your shoulders. Walk to the opposite cone and return to your starting point, keeping the dumbbells in this position while maintaining a strong, upright posture.

6 FRONT SQUAT

Stand next to one cone with your feet shoulder-width apart and hold the lighter dumbbells in each hand at your shoulders with your elbows directly underneath the handles of the dumbbells (see figure g). Squat as low as you can by bending your knees and sitting your hips back (see figure h); do not allow your heels to rise off the floor or allow your lower back to round out. Reverse the motion and return to the tall standing position to complete 1 rep. Perform 8 to 10 reps total.

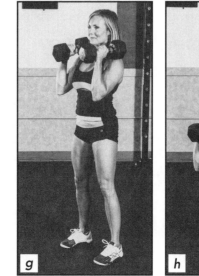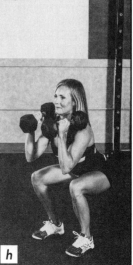

7 FARMER'S WALK

As described previously, stand next to one cone and hold two heavy dumbbells on each side of your body, with palms facing the body, either by your hips or at your shoulders. Walk to the opposite cone and return to your starting point, keeping the dumbbells in this position while maintaining a strong, upright posture.

Unilateral Farmer's Walk Complex

This complex is performed in the same fashion as the bilateral farmer's walk, except you do the entire complex using the same side. You'll first perform this complex on the left side, then you'll rest, and then you'll repeat it on your right side. Following are the exercises for this complex.

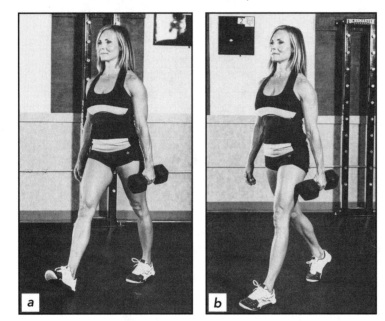

1 ONE-ARM FARMER'S WALK

Stand next to one cone and hold a heavy dumbbell on one side of your body, with your palm facing your body, either by your hip or at your shoulder (see figure a for an example at the hip). Walk to the opposite cone and return to your starting point, keeping the dumbbell in this position while maintaining a strong upright posture (see figure b).

2 FREESTANDING ONE-ARM ROW

Stand next to one cone and stand in a split stance with your right leg in front of your left leg and with both knees slightly bent, holding a lighter dumbbell with your left hand. Hinge at your hips, keeping your back straight so that your torso becomes parallel with the floor (see figure c). Perform a row, pulling the dumbbell toward your body without rotating the shoulders or hips, making sure to pull your scapula toward your spine in a controlled manner as your arm moves into your body (see figure d). Be sure to maintain a stable spinal position, keeping your back straight throughout the exercise. Slowly lower the dumbbell toward the floor without letting it touch the floor to complete 1 rep. Perform 10 to 12 reps total.

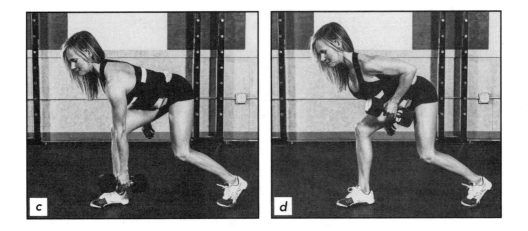

❸ ONE-ARM FARMER'S WALK

As described previously, stand next to one cone and hold a heavy dumbbell on one side of your body, with your palm facing your body, either by your hip or at your shoulder. Walk to the opposite cone and return to your starting point, keeping the dumbbell in this position while maintaining a strong upright posture.

❹ ONE-ARM OVERHEAD PRESS

Stand next to one cone with your feet roughly shoulder-width apart and hold a lighter dumbbell at shoulder level (see figure e). Press the dumbbell toward the sky, keeping your torso as stable as possible (see figure f). Slowly lower the dumbbell to your shoulder. Perform 10 to 12 reps total.

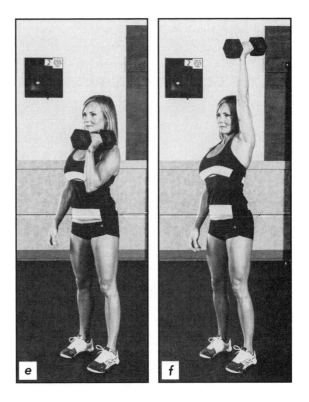

❺ ONE-ARM FARMER'S WALK

As described previously, stand next to one cone and hold a heavy dumbbell on one side of your body, with your palm facing your body, either by your hip or at your shoulder. Walk to the opposite cone and return to your starting point, keeping the dumbbell in this position while maintaining a strong upright posture.

6 REVERSE LUNGE WITH DUMBBELL AT SHOULDER

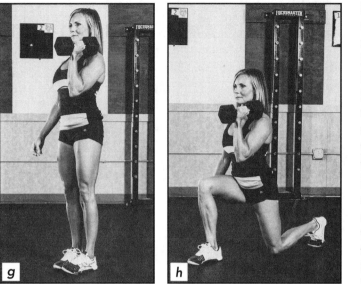

Stand next to one cone with your feet about hip-width apart and hold a lighter dumbbell in your left hand at your shoulder (see figure g). Step backward with your left foot and drop your body so your knee lightly touches the floor (see figure h). Reverse the movement by coming out of the lunge and bringing your foot forward so that you are back to your starting position. Perform these reverse lunges by only stepping back with this one leg. Stepping back with this leg while holding the dumbbell in the same-side hand forces you to work your one leg, which keeps you better balanced and feels more natural than if you stepped back with your other leg. Perform 10 to 12 reps total.

7 ONE-ARM FARMER'S WALK

As described previously, stand next to one cone and hold a heavy dumbbell on one side of your body, with your palm facing your body, either by your hip or at your shoulder. Walk to the opposite cone and return to your starting point, keeping the dumbbell in this position while maintaining a strong upright posture.

Plate Push Complex

A plate complex involves a 45-pound weight plate and a pair of dumbbells. It's a series of dumbbell exercises alternating with several sets of weight-plate pushes. These complexes are performed back to back (circuit style) without rest until all exercises within a given complex have been completed. A basketball court or track surface is ideal for the plate push.

Plate Push Complex 1

Perform 2 to 4 sets with 2 to 4 minutes of rest between sets. Following are the exercises for this complex.

1 BENT-OVER ROW

Stand with your feet roughly hip-width apart. Hold a lighter dumbbell in each hand using a neutral grip so your palms are facing one another, keeping your hands just outside shoulder-width apart. Bend over at your hips, keeping your back straight so that your torso is parallel to the floor and your knees are bent 15 to 20 degrees (see figure *a*). Row the dumbbells into your sides at belly-button level (see figure *b*). Slowly lower the dumbbells until your arms are straight to complete 1 rep. Perform 6 to 8 reps total.

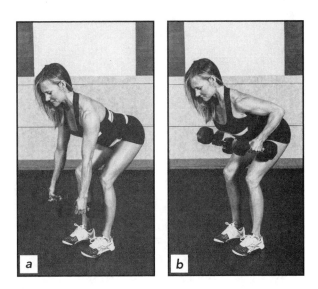

2 PLATE PUSH

Place a 25-, 35-, or 45-pound Olympic plate on top of a towel to create a slippery surface. You can also place dumbbells on top of the weight-plate to further increase the load. Place your hands on the center of the weight-plate or on the dumbbells and assume a push-up position. Driving with your legs, push the plate 20 to 25 yards as fast as you can down the court or track surface and back (see figures *c* and *d*). When performing a plate push, keep your back straight, avoid lifting your hips higher than your shoulders, and keep your arms and elbows straight throughout the exercise. Also take long strides, pushing your legs hard into the ground with each step.

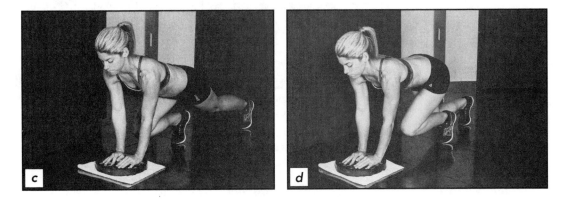

3 OVERHEAD PRESS

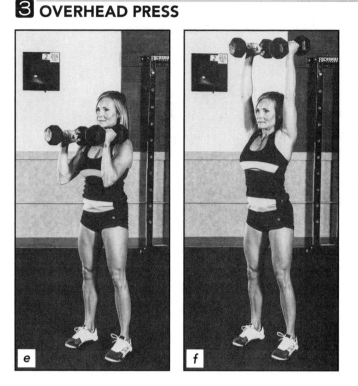

Stand tall with your feet roughly shoulder-width apart while holding a dumbbell in each hand at shoulder level (see figure e). Push both dumbbells overhead keeping your torso as stable as possible (see figure f). Slowly lower the dumbbells back to your shoulders.

4 PLATE PUSH

As described previously, perform a plate push for another 20 to 25 yards down the court or track surface and back.

5 ONE-LEG ROMANIAN DEADLIFT

Stand on your right leg, holding a dumbbell in each hand (see figure g). Keeping your back and both arms straight, hinge at your hip and bend forward toward the floor, keeping your right knee bent at roughly a 15- to 20-degree angle (see figure h). As you hinge,

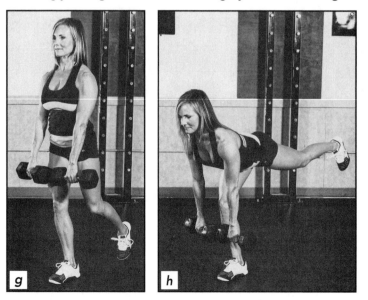

allow your non-weight-bearing leg to elevate so it remains in a straight line with your torso while also not allowing your lower back to round out. At the bottom position (when your torso is roughly parallel to the ground), be sure to keep your hips flat and do not allow them to rotate. Once your torso and non-weight-bearing leg are roughly parallel to the floor, reverse the motion by driving your hips forward to stand tall again and complete 1 rep. Switch your stance leg on each rep. Perform 10 to 12 total reps.

6 PLATE PUSH

As described previously, perform a plate push for another 20 to 25 yards down the court or track surface and back.

7 PUSH-UP TO PLANK ROW

Assume a plank push-up position with one hand on the handle of each dumbbell, directly under your shoulders (see figure *i*). Perform a push-up by lowering your body to the floor while keeping your elbows directly above your wrists the entire time (see figure *j*). Once your ribs come in contact with the dumbbells, reverse the motion by pushing your body up (see figure *k*). Do not allow your head or hips to sag toward the floor at any time. From the top of push-up position, row the left dumbbell up into your body until it touches your left ribs (see figure *l*). Slowly lower the dumbbell back to the floor and row the left dumbbell in the same manner. While rowing the dumbbells, be sure your torso remains as stable as possible; do not allow your hips to rotate at any time. Perform 6 to 8 reps total.

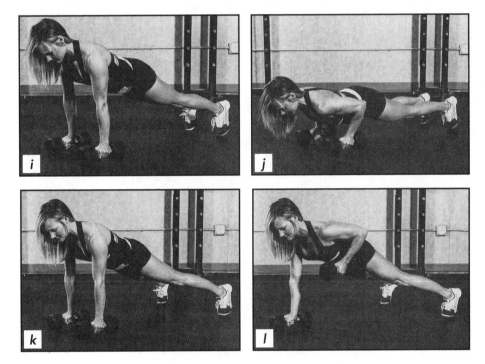

Plate Push Complex 2

Perform 2 to 4 sets with 2 to 4 minutes of rest between sets. Following are the exercises for this complex.

1 UPPERCUT

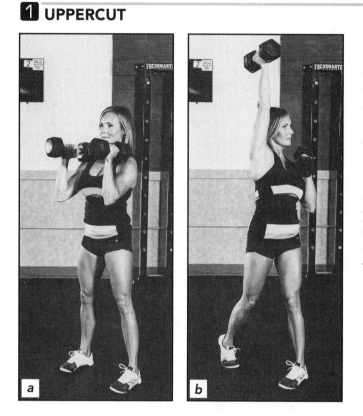

Stand tall with your feet roughly shoulder-width apart while holding a dumbbell in front of each shoulder (see figure a). Press one dumbbell into the air as you rotate to the opposite side (see figure b). Reverse the motion and repeat while rotating to the other side. To better allow your hips to rotate in this exercise, allow your heel to come off the ground as you turn. Perform 6 to 10 total reps.

2 PLATE PUSH

Place a 25-, 35-, or 45-pound Olympic plate on top of a towel to create a slippery surface. You can also place dumbbells on top of the weight-plate to further increase the load. Place your hands on the center of the weight-plate or on the dumbbells and assume a push-up position. Driving with your legs, push the plate 20 to 25 yards as fast as you can down the court or track surface and back (see figures c and d). When performing a plate push, keep your back straight, avoid lifting your hips higher than your shoulders, and keep your arms and elbows straight throughout the exercise. Also take long strides, pushing your legs hard into the ground with each step.

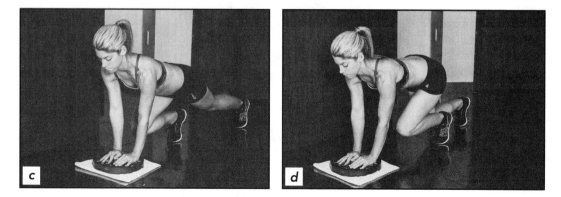

3 HIGH PULL

Stand with your feet hip-width apart and hold a dumbbell in each hand. Slightly hinge at your hips and slightly bend your knees (see figure *e*). Explosively drive your hips and knee straight while simultaneously pulling the dumbbells up, keeping your elbows pointing upward (see figure *f*). Once the dumbbells reach chest level, lower them to the starting position. Perform 6 to 8 reps total.

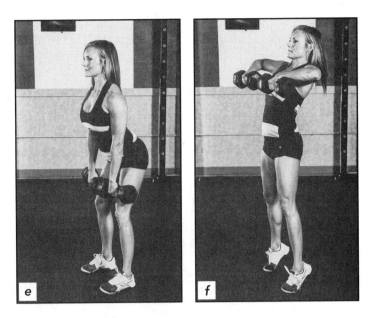

4 PLATE PUSH

As described previously, perform a plate push for another 20 yards down the court or track surface and back.

5 ONE-LEG ROMANIAN DEADLIFT

Stand on your right leg, holding a dumbbell in each hand (see figure *g*). Keeping your back and both arms straight, hinge at your hip and bend forward toward the floor, keeping your right knee bent at roughly a 15- to 20-degree angle (see figure *h*). As you hinge, allow your non-weight-bearing leg to elevate so it remains in a straight line with your torso while also

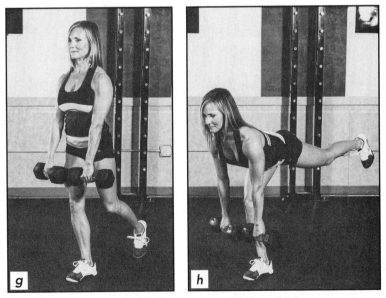

not allowing your lower back to round out. At the bottom position (when your torso is roughly parallel to the ground), be sure to keep your hips flat and do not allow them to rotate. Once your torso and non-weight-bearing leg are roughly parallel to the floor, reverse the motion by driving your hips forward to stand tall again and complete 1 rep. Switch your stance leg on each rep. Perform 10 to 12 total reps.

6 PLATE PUSH

As described previously, perform a plate push for another 20 yards down the court or track surface and back.

7 BREAK-DANCER PUSH-UP

Begin in a push-up position with your hands and feet shoulder-width apart (see figure *i*). Perform a push-up, and at the top of the repetition, rotate your entire body toward your left side, driving your right knee to your left elbow while keeping your left hand in contact with your chin (see figure *j*). Reverse this motion to perform another push-up and repeat this action on the opposite side, touching your left knee to your right elbow. Perform 10 to 20 reps total.

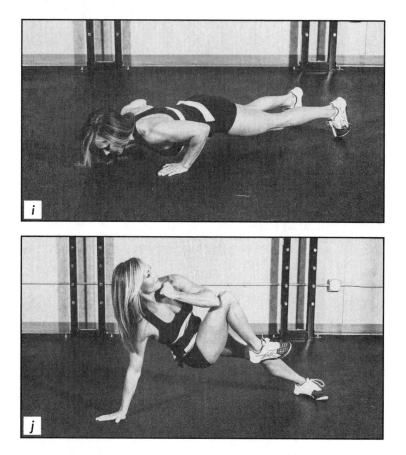

The beauty of the metabolic strength training complexes featured in this chapter, along with the protocols featured in the body-weight training chapter, is that they've all been carefully designed to allow you to flow seamlessly from one exercise to the other. This not only makes them easier to memorize but also more effective to use because they allow you to get a lot of high-quality exercise done while integrating a wide variety of movements into a short amount of time. This yields big results in accelerating your metabolism and helping you maintain muscle.

Body-Weight Training

Whether you have a gym membership or not, you can't always make it to the gym. That's okay, because this chapter is all about exercises that can help you shed body fat while becoming stronger and more athletic using the best piece of exercise equipment ever invented—the human body. These body-weight training concepts will help you develop a world-class workout that improves your strength and increases your metabolism at a moment's notice—wherever you are!

Contrary to popular belief, body-weight training is not just for beginners, nor is it limited to basic moves such as push-ups and squats. As with the rest of the practical exercise chapters in this book, the exercise concepts in this chapter feature basic to advanced training applications that will challenge even the most elite athlete. You'll also probably learn some new body-weight moves and protocols you've never tried before.

PROS AND CONS OF BODY-WEIGHT TRAINING

Anyone from elite athletes to beginning exercisers can benefit from the body-weight training concepts in this chapter. Here's a list of the advantages of body-weight training.

It's Space Efficient

An effective body-weight workout can be performed in an area the size of an elevator. This can help when you're training at home, on the go, or in a crowed gym. Forget about waiting for machines and dealing the crowded weight areas. With these body-weight training moves, your body is your weight machine!

It's Travel Friendly

Body-weight training is an essential tool for working professionals who are in and out of hotels. No space, no gym, no problem!

It Focuses on Natural Movement

Body-weight exercises allow your body to move how it wants to and follow its most comfortable patterns of action. This can be valuable in gaining athleticism by improving body awareness.

It Builds Relative Body Strength

Relative body strength is how strong you are relative to your own body weight and how capable you are of controlling your body weight without additional load. This can also aid in improving athleticism and improving body awareness in sports, because in most sports you use only your body weight and don't carry around external loads.

However, there's no reason to *only* use body-weight training. Keep in mind the saying, "Master your body with body-weight training. Master your environment with external loads." In other words, don't exclusively use body-weight training if you have access to free weights and weight machines. Free weights (e.g., dumbbells, barbells, resistance bands, machines) offer unique benefits, and using all of the modalities in conjunction with each other will yield better results than exclusively using only one modality.

Another reason it's not a great idea to limit yourself exclusively to body-weight training is because it severely limits the exercise options for strengthening your back (i.e., pulling) muscles. You must have something to pull yourself up to, such as a chin-up bar (and many beginners cannot do chin-ups even if they have a bar), or you must have something you can pull on, such as heavy-duty resistance bands. Without these, the options for creating a balanced strength training program by using a variety of pulling exercises to offset all of the body-weight push-up options are virtually nonexistent. For this reason, if you often train at home or in hotel rooms, your best option is to buy a chin-up bar for home use and a set of high-quality resistance bands for both home use and to take with you when you travel. These bands are very portable and can be attached to any doorway or stable object in matter of seconds. They come in multiple resistances from light to very heavy and add a tremendous number of effective exercise options to your body-weight training workouts, delivering a value that far exceeds their cost. (As you'll see later in this chapter, we cover many pulling exercises using resistance bands and also a suspension trainer.)

The goal of this chapter is to offer body-weight exercises you can use to get a gym-quality workout when you can't get to the gym. In the workouts chapter of this book, you'll find several workouts that integrate many of the body-weight protocols from this chapter with exercises from other chapters that use equipment in order to create a more comprehensive, interesting, and well-rounded workout. For times when you don't have access to the gym, workout programs are also provided that exclusively use the exercises in this chapter.

BODY-WEIGHT EXERCISES

Following you'll find exercise applications that can be integrated into a circuit. You'll also find exercise combinations and complexes to give you effective options for each of the three Cs. Additionally, some of the exercise applications use a stability ball, which is an inexpensive training tool that enhances your body-weight workouts at home or on the go.

Body-Weight Leg Exercises

With the right exercises, sometimes your own body weight is all you need to strengthen your legs and build a well-balanced lower body that won't quit. Speaking of well balanced, you'll notice that most of the lower-body exercises in this chapter are unilateral. This is due to the fact that most of us have one leg that isn't as strong or as well developed as the other, and single-leg exercises are the optimal way to improve your muscle balance. They are also an effective way to increase the workload on your lower-body muscles without having to hold extra loads such as a barbell or dumbbells. Instead of both of your legs splitting the weight of your upper body evenly, single-leg training doubles the load that each leg experiences, because each leg is forced to move the weight of your entire body by itself. Following are a variety of lower-body leg-oriented exercises using body weight.

PRISONER SQUAT

Stand tall with your feet shoulder-width apart and your toes turned out slightly, about 10 degrees. Interlace your fingers behind your head with your elbows pointing out to the sides (see figure *a*). Perform a squat by bending your knees and sitting back at your hips (see figure *b*). Go as low as you can possibly go without allowing your lower back to round out. Be sure that as you squat you do not allow your heels to come off the ground or your knees to come together toward the midline of your body. Your knees should track in the same direction as your toes.

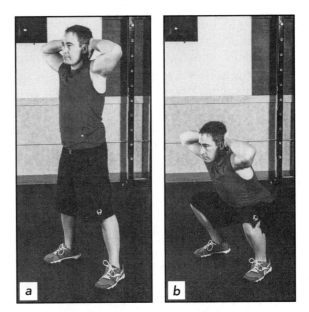

PRISONER REVERSE LUNGE

Stand with your feet hip-width apart and your fingers interlaced behind your head with your elbows pointing out to the sides (see figure *a*). Step backward with your left foot and drop your body so your knee lightly touches the floor (see figure *b*). Reverse the movement by coming out of the lunge and bringing your left foot forward so that you are back to your starting position. Perform the same movement on the opposite leg.

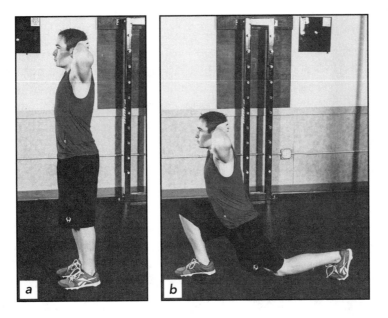

KNEE-TAP SQUAT

The only difference between body-weight knee-tap squats and the version using dumbbells you learned in chapter 4 is the positioning of your arms.

Bend one knee 90 degrees and hold it slightly behind your weight-bearing leg with your arms outstretched in front of you (see figure a). Squat until your back knee lightly taps a small platform on the floor behind you (see figure b) and reverse the motion to complete 1 repetition. Be sure to keep your weight-bearing foot completely flat throughout this exercise. You can remove the platform and touch your knee to the floor. Also, due to the increased range of motion, you'll have to lean your torso slightly forward at the bottom position. This is okay when working with just body weight because the load on your back is minimal, unlike when you're holding dumbbells.

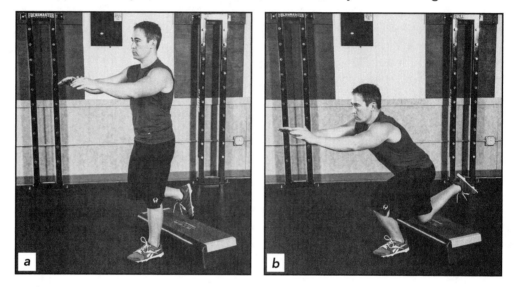

PRISONER CYCLE LUNGE

Stand tall with your feet together and with your fingers interlaced behind your head (see figure a). Step forward with your left leg and drop into a lunge (see figure b). Then reverse the motion by stepping into a reverse lunge with your left leg to complete 1 rep (see figure c). Repeat all reps using the same leg before switching sides.

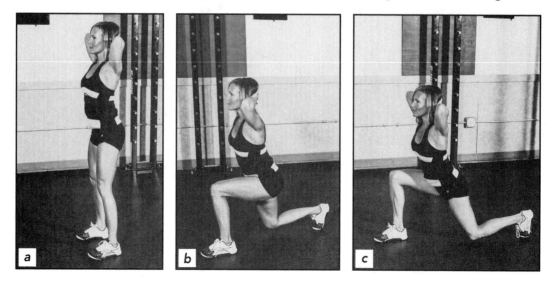

PRISONER SQUAT JUMP

Stand tall with your feet shoulder-width apart and your toes turned out slightly, about 10 degrees. Interlace your fingers behind your head with your elbows pointing out to the sides. Perform a squat by bending your knees and sitting back at your hips (see figure a). Go as low as you can possibly go without allowing your lower back to round out. As you squat down, be sure that you do not allow your heels to come off the ground or your knees to come together toward the midline. Your knees should track in the same direction as your toes. Quickly

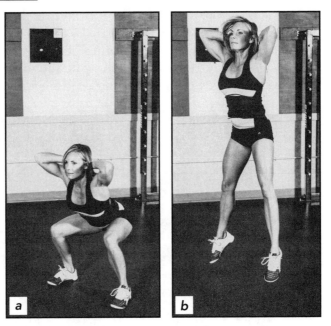

reverse the motion, jumping into the air as high as you can (see figure b). Land as lightly as possible back into the bottom of the squat position.

LATERAL LUNGE

Stand tall with your arms outstretched in front of you at shoulder level (see figure a). Take a big step to one side, dropping your hips to that same side while keeping both feet flat and your spine straight (see figure b). Quickly reverse the motion, bringing your feet back together. You can either perform all reps on one side or alternate legs.

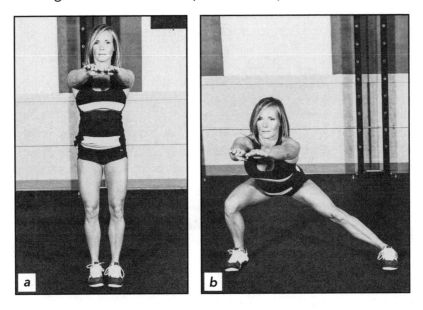

ROTATIONAL LUNGE

Stand tall with your arms outstretched in front of you at shoulder level (see figure *a*). Take a big step 45 degrees behind you, dropping your hips to that same side while keeping your foot flat on the lunging side and your trailing leg straight (see figure *b*). Quickly reverse the motion, bringing your feet back together. You can either perform all reps on one side or alternate legs.

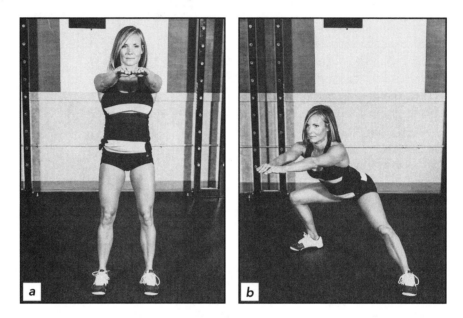

SPLIT-SQUAT SCISSOR JUMP

From a split stance with your fingers interlaced behind your head (see figure *a*), jump into the air, scissoring your legs (see figure *b*) so that you land with the opposite leg forward (see figure *c*). Jump into the air again, repeating this action. Be sure to land as quietly and as lightly as possible, using each landing to load the next jump.

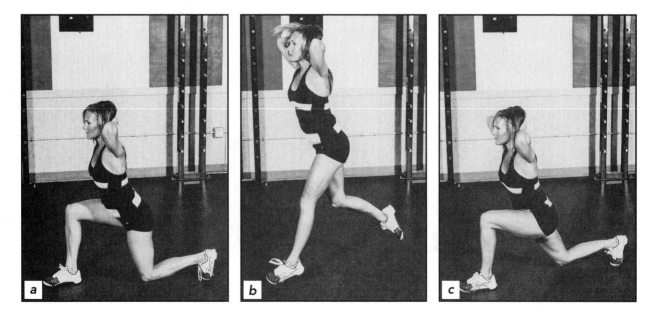

OVERHEAD WALKING LUNGE

Stand tall with your arms extended straight overhead in line with your torso and with your feet hip-width apart (see figure a). Take a large step forward and drop your body so your back knee lightly touches the floor (see figure b). Stand up tall again while simultaneously bringing your rear leg forward to meet your front leg (see figure c). Step forward with the opposite leg (the one that was behind you on the last rep). A slight forward torso lean with a straight spine instead of an upright torso at the bottom of each lunge is okay; it's a bit easier on your knees because the slight forward lean will help recruit your glutes. Repeat as you move down the room.

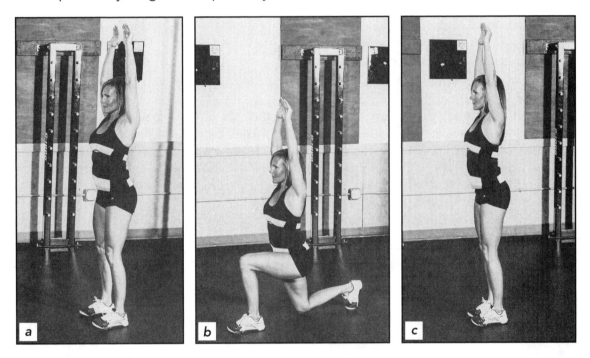

OVERHEAD REVERSE LUNGE

This is a great lunge option if you have limited training space because the mechanics are the same as in the walking lunge, except you don't move across the room and you step backward instead of forward. With your arms extended above your head and with your feet hip-width apart, step backward with one foot and drop your body so your knee lightly touches the floor (see figure a). Reverse the movement by coming out of the lunge and bringing your same foot forward so that you are back to your starting position (see figure b). Perform the same movement on the opposite leg.

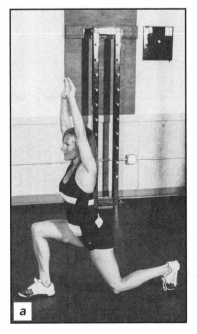
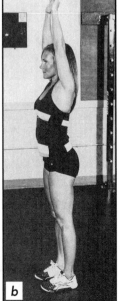

Body-Weight Hip Exercises

These days it's not uncommon to sit for several hours, whether you are at work or at home on your computer, and when you sit, the muscles of your posterior hips, the glutes, are in a lengthened position. This can eventually cause them to adapt and become weaker at doing their job, which is to extend your hips—the opposite of the position your hips are in when you're sitting. Here are several body-weight hip exercises that can help you reverse the negative effects of the sitting position. In addition, they can give you a body that not only looks better but also performs better, because the glutes are a primary source of power when it comes to running faster and jumping higher.

ONE-LEG HIP THRUST

From position with your shoulders elevated on a weight bench or chair, rest your head and shoulders on the bench and open your arms to the sides with palms facing up. Walk your legs out until your knees are bent at about 90 degrees and your feet are directly below your knees. Keeping your right knee bent 90 degrees, lift it above your hip (see figure a). Lift your hips so that your body makes a straight line from knees to nose (see figure b). Keeping your right leg lifted, lower your hips toward the floor, and then press your hips back up through your left heel to complete each rep. You can make this move more difficult by adding weight—try holding a weighted bar across your hips. Perform all reps on the same side before switching to the other leg.

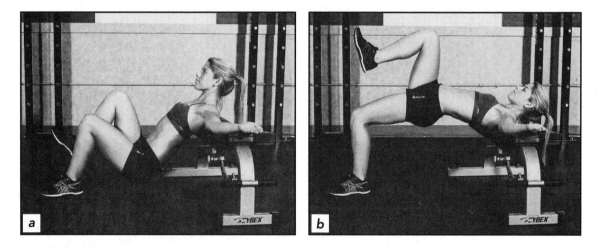

STABILITY-BALL LEG CURL

Lie in a supine position on the floor with your heels resting on top of a 55- to 65-centimeter stability ball and your arms out to the sides for balance (see figure a). Raise your hips toward the sky while simultaneously pulling your heels toward your body underneath you (see figure b). Slowly reverse the motion and repeat without allowing your hips to touch the floor. To perform a single-leg variation, simply raise one leg off the ball, flexing your hip and knee at a 90-degree angle, and perform the same action as described. Complete all the repetitions on one side before switching to the other leg.

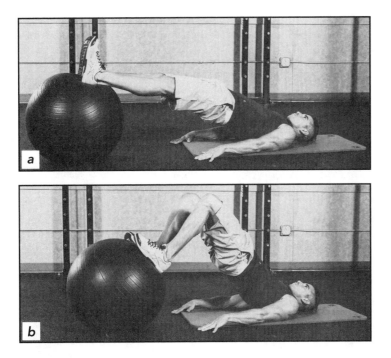

STABILITY-BALL HIP LIFT

Lie in a supine position with your knees bent 15 degrees and your feet on top of a 55- to 65-centimeter stability ball (see figure *a*). Raise your hips into the air, extending from your hips, not your lower back (see figure *b*). Slowly lower your hips until just before they touch the floor and repeat. To perform this exercise using one leg, simply follow the same action with one hip and knee flexed at a 90-degree angle. Complete all the repetitions on one side before switching to the other leg.

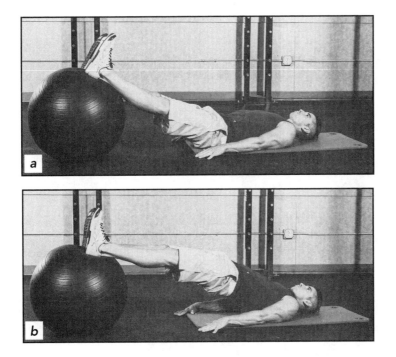

ANTERIOR-LEANING LUNGE SCISSOR JUMP

This action is performed in the same manner as the split-squat scissor jump described earlier, only in this exercise your torso position is angled forward. From a split stance with your arms by your sides (see figure *a*), jump into the air, scissoring your legs (see figure *b*) so that you land with the opposite leg forward (see figure *c*). Jump into the air again, repeating this action. Be sure to land as quietly and as lightly as possible, using each landing to load the next jump. Each time you land, hinge forward at your hips, keeping your spine straight so that your hands reach down by your ankles. Each time you explode back into the air, raise your torso.

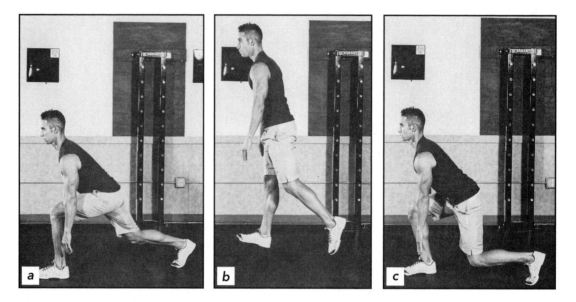

LATERAL BOUND

Balance on your left leg with your right leg held off the ground by bending your knee and lifting your heel behind you (see figure *a*). While reaching across your body with your right arm, squat down and explode toward your right side, jumping as far you can (see figure *b*). Land softly on your right leg in a single-leg squat position, reaching across your body with your left arm (see figure *c*). Then repeat by jumping back to the left side. Be sure to land with a soft knee into a squat position to ensure maximal force absorption and power production on the next jump.

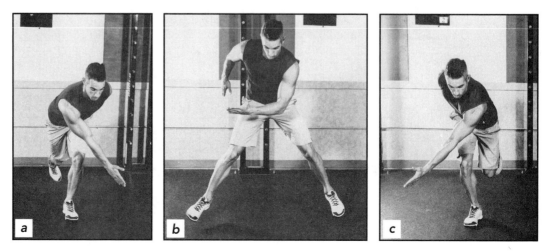

FROG JUMP

With your knees bent roughly 20 degrees, hinge forward at your hips so that your back is parallel to the floor and your fingertips touch the ground in between your legs (see figure a). With a straight spine, explode into the air, straightening your body in midair (see figure b). Land as softly as possible in the starting position and repeat the jump.

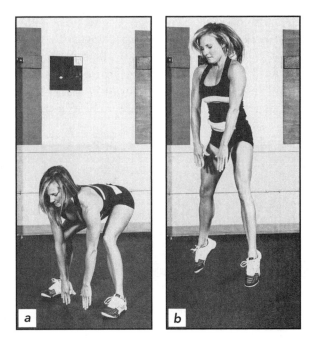

BULGARIAN SPLIT SQUAT

Interlace your fingers behind your head and assume a split-squat stance by placing one foot on top of a bench or chair that's behind you (see figure a). Lower your body toward the floor without allowing your back knee to rest on the floor (see figure b). As you lower your body, keep your back straight and lean your torso slightly forward. Drive your heel into the ground to raise your body back to the starting position to complete 1 rep. Perform all reps on one side before switching legs.

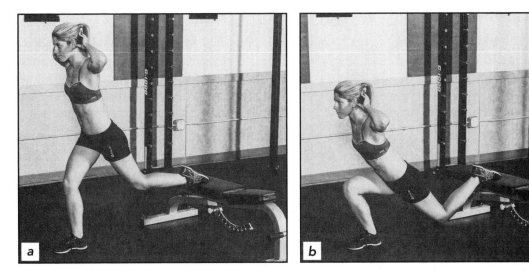

ONE-LEG GOOD MORNING

Balance on one leg with your hands above your head (see figure a). With your weight-bearing knee bent 20 degrees, hinge at your hip, keeping your back straight and your arms in line with your torso until your body (including your non-weight-bearing leg) is parallel with the floor (see figure b). Be sure to keep your hips and rear foot from rotating by keeping your shoulders and hips flat throughout the exercise. Perform all reps on one side before switching legs.

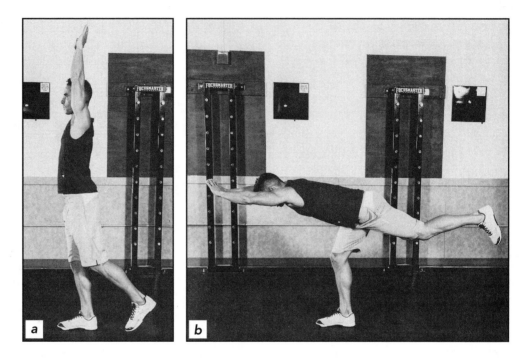

Upper-Body Body-Weight Pushing Exercises

It should be no secret that when it comes to body-weight training, the push-up is going be involved. That being said, the following exercises include several push-up variations, some of which may be a new twist on this classic exercise. In addition to some unique push-up variations, you will also find some band exercises designed to work the upper-body pushing muscles (chest, shoulders, triceps) and core musculature.

ONE-ARM PUSH-UP

Assume a one-arm plank position with your feet spread several inches wider than your shoulders (see figure a). Your weight-bearing arm should be positioned so that your wrist is directly under your same-side shoulder. Your non-weight-bearing arm should be on your same-side hip. Drop into a one-arm push-up without allowing your torso to rotate while keeping your elbow on the working side tight to your body (see figure b). Drive into the floor and push your body back to the top of the push-up to complete 1 rep. Perform all repetitions on one side before switching to the other arm.

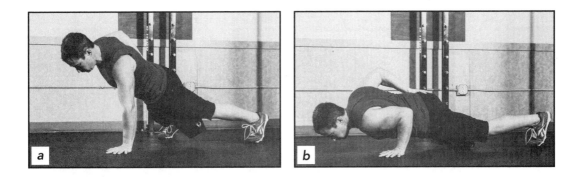

PUSH-UP LOCK-OFF

Begin in a push-up position with one hand on top of a medicine ball or platform and your other hand on the floor with your feet shoulder-width apart. Perform a push-up with one hand on top of the platform or medicine ball (see figure *a*). At the top of the push-up, lock off by fully straightening the elbow of the arm that's resting on the platform or medicine ball without allowing your shoulders or hips to rotate. Place the other arm at the chest (see figure *b*). Perform half of the repetitions with your right arm elevated and the other half with your left arm elevated.

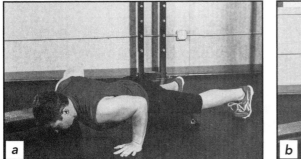
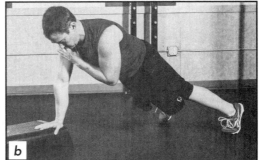

BOX CROSSOVER PUSH-UP

Begin in a push-up position with both hands on top of a medicine ball or platform and your feet shoulder-width apart (see figure *a*). Step one hand off the box or ball to the floor while performing a push-up (see figure *b*). As you come out of the push-up, bring your hand back to the platform or ball. Repeat the same action to the other side.

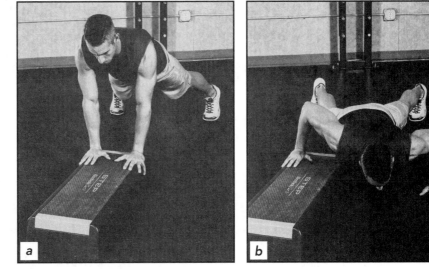

BREAK-DANCER PUSH-UP

Begin in a push-up position with your hands and feet shoulder-width apart. Perform a push-up (see figure *a*), and at the top of the repetition, rotate your entire body toward your left side, driving your right knee to your left elbow while keeping your left hand either in front of your face or against your jaw (see figure *b*). Reverse this motion to perform another push-up and repeat this action on the opposite side, touching your left knee to your right elbow.

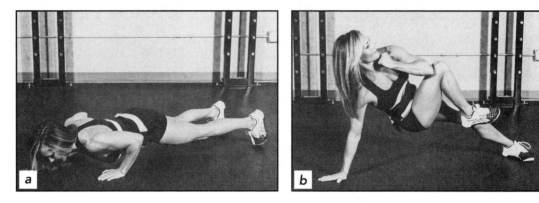

PUSH-BACK PUSH-UP

Begin in a push-up position with your hands and feet shoulder-width apart (see figure *a*), then drop into the bottom of the push-up (see figure *b*). Instead of pushing up out of the push-up in the traditional manner, soften your knees and push yourself backward toward your feet, keeping your hips as low as possible (see figure *c*). Reverse this motion and drop into the bottom of the push-up to complete 1 rep.

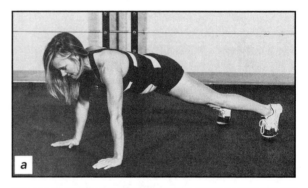

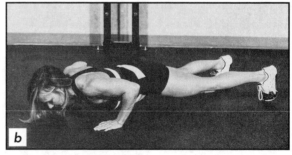

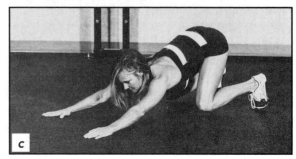

PUSH-BACK PUSH-UP WITH TWIST

This is a more-advanced version of the push-back push-up that is performed in basically the same manner as described in the previous exercise. Begin in a push-up position with your hands and feet shoulder-width apart (see figure a). Then drop into the bottom push-up position (see figure b). Instead of pushing up out of the push-up in the traditional manner, soften your knees and push yourself backward toward your feet, keeping your hips as low as possible and twisting your body so as to put all of your weight onto one arm (see figure c and d). Reverse this motion, place your elevated hand back onto to the floor, and drop into the bottom of another push-up, this time finishing by twisting your body to the other side and lifting your other arm off of the floor.

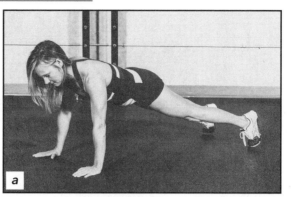

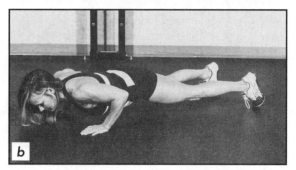

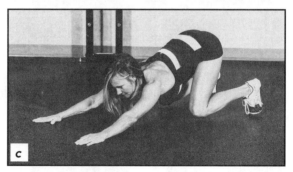

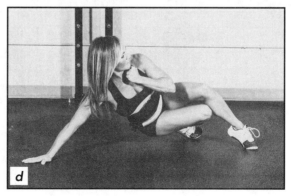

FEET-ELEVATED PUSH-UP

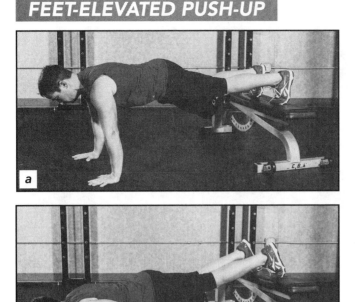

Begin in a push-up position with your hands on the floor just wider than shoulder-width apart and with your feet elevated on top of a weight bench or chair (see figure a). Perform a push-up by lowering your chest toward the floor until your elbows reach just below 90 degrees (see figure b). Then press yourself away from the floor until your elbows are straight. Be sure to keep your body in a straight line from your head to your hips to your ankles and do not allow your head or hips to sag toward the floor at any time.

LUNGE AND BAND PRESS

Face away from a band that's attached at roughly shoulder height to a stable structure or inside a doorjamb (many resistance bands come with an attachment for this). With your feet hip-width apart and in a parallel stance, hold a handle in each hand, with your elbows out to your sides and your forearms parallel to the floor (see figure a). Lunge forward while simultaneously performing a chest press with both arms, adding a slight lean forward to bring in your abdominal muscles (see figure b). Step back to the starting position, allowing your arms to come back as well. Repeat the press while lunging forward with the other leg.

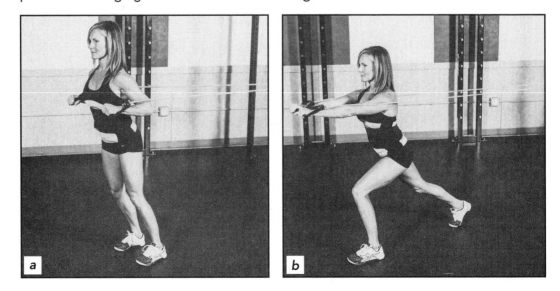

ONE-ARM BAND PRESS

Face away from a band that's attached at roughly shoulder height to a stable structure or inside a doorjamb (many resistance bands come with an attachment for this). Stand in a split stance with your right leg in front and hold both handles of the band in your left hand (see figure *a*). Without allowing your torso to rotate, drive your arm straight out in front of you (see figure *b*). Slowly bring your arm back to complete 1 rep. Perform all reps on one side before switching arms and reversing your stance.

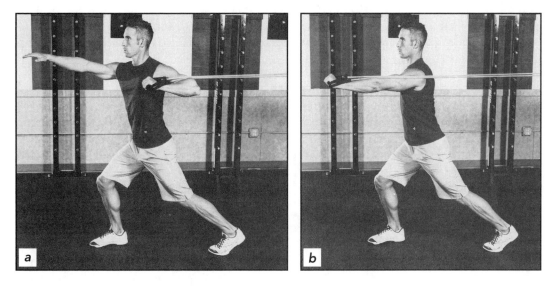

ONE-ARM INCLINE BAND PRESS

Face away from a band that's attached at a low position (below knee level) to a stable structure or inside a doorjamb (many resistance bands come with an attachment for this). Stand in a split stance with your right leg in front and hold both handles of the band in your left hand (see figure *a*). Without allowing your torso to rotate, drive your arm straight out at a 45-degree angle (see figure *b*). Be sure to keep your arm at the same angle as the band. Slowly bring your arm back to complete 1 rep. Perform all reps on one side before switching arms and reversing your stance.

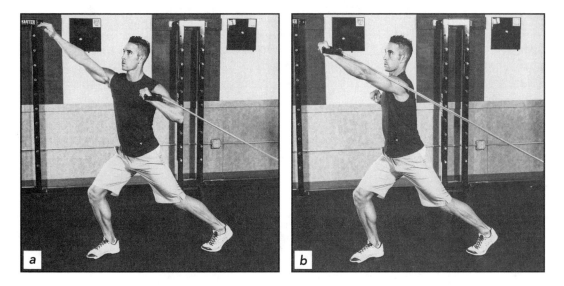

SUSPENSION TRICEPS SKULL CRUSHER

Facing away from the anchor point, grab onto the handles and lean your weight forward in a push-up position with your arms extended directly in front of your shoulders (see figure a). Bend at your elbows and lower your forehead to your wrists (see figure b). Reverse the direction and extend your elbows as in a triceps extension to complete 1 rep.

Be sure to keep your entire body straight throughout the action. To increase the difficulty, lower your body closer to the floor. The closer your shoulders come to being under the anchor point, the tougher the exercise becomes. To decrease the difficulty, assume a higher angle position. The farther your feet are in front of the anchor point, the easier the exercise becomes.

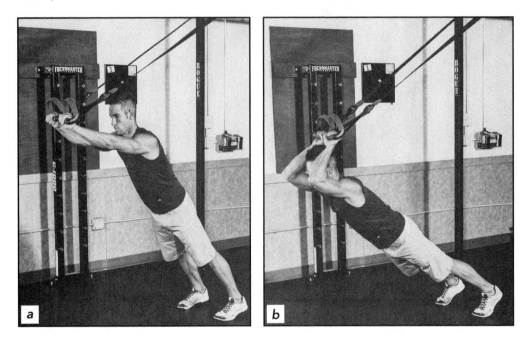

Upper-Body Body-Weight Pulling Exercises

As valuable and versatile as body-weight training is, its biggest limitation is upper-body pulling exercises. Of course there are pull-ups and chin-ups, but many people have a difficult time with these. This is why both a suspension trainer and a set of resistance bands are used in the body-weight exercises featured in this chapter. These affordable and versatile pieces of equipment not only give you all the benefits of a cable machine, they also allow you to balance all of your upper-body pushing work with several valuable pulling options to strengthen the muscles of the back, shoulders, biceps, and core.

CHIN-UP OR PULL-UP

Hang from a bar with either a parallel, underhand grip, or wide grip (see figure a for an example using an overhand grip). Pull yourself up to the bar as powerfully as possible (see figure b) and then lower yourself in a slow and controlled manner, allowing no momentum or swinging.

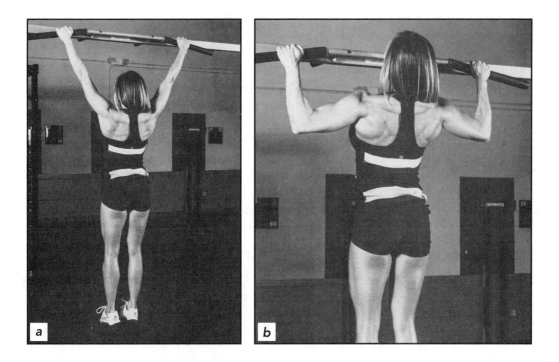

SINGLE-ARM ANTIROTATION SUSPENSION ROW

Facing the anchor point of a suspension trainer and holding a handle in your right hand, lean backward so your feet are roughly underneath the anchor point and extend your left arm by your side (see figure *a*). Without allowing your body to rotate at any point, perform rows by pulling your body toward the handle (see figure *b*) and lowering back down, keeping your elbow (on the rowing side) tight to your body each time you pull yourself toward the handle. Do not allow your hips to sag toward the floor, and be sure to keep your shoulders and hips parallel to the floor through the entire exercise. To increase the difficulty, walk your feet farther in to increase your body angle and bring you lower to the floor. To decrease the difficulty, decrease your body angle by walking your feet in so they're more underneath you.

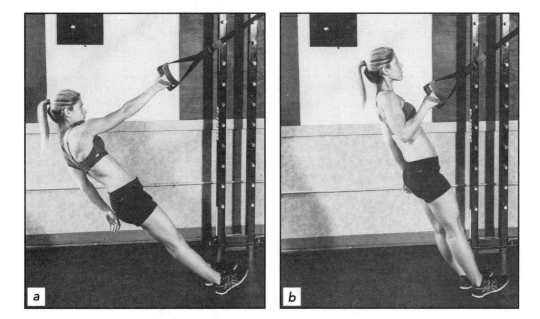

LOW-ELBOW SUSPENSION ROW

Face the anchor point of the suspension trainer. Hold onto the handles with your palms either facing each other or the sky and with your arms straight and extended in front of your shoulders (see figure a for an example with palms facing each other). Lean back with your body in a straight line from head to toe. Pull yourself up toward your hands by bending at your elbows and performing a rowing motion (see figure b). Be sure to keep your body in a straight line and do not lead with your hips when pulling yourself up. Touch the insides of your wrists to your bottom ribs with each row to ensure a full range of motion, and keep your elbows tight to your sides. Pause at the top for a 1- to 2-second hold before returning to the starting position to complete 1 rep. To increase the difficulty, start the exercise from a more severe backward lean, bringing your body closer to the floor.

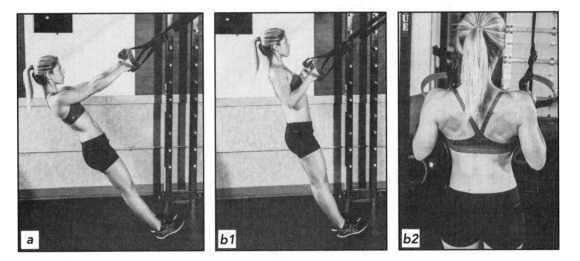

WIDE-ELBOW SUSPENSION ROW

With your body facing the anchor point of the suspension trainer, hold onto the handles with your thumbs facing each other and your arms straight and extended out in front of your shoulders (see figure a). Lean back with your body in a straight line from head to toe. Pull yourself up toward your hands by bending at your elbows and performing a rowing motion while flaring out your elbows (see figure b). Be sure to keep your body in a straight line and do not lead with your hips when pulling yourself up.

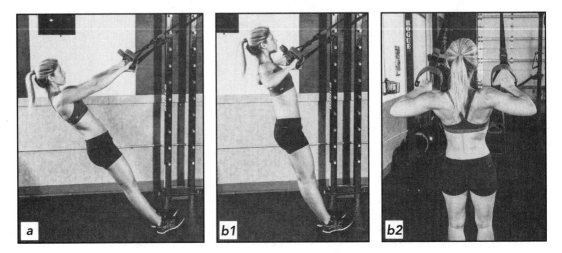

Your elbows will form a 90-degree angle. Pause at the top for a 1- to 2-second hold before returning to the starting position to complete 1 rep. To increase the difficulty, start the exercise from a more severe backward lean, bringing your body closer to the floor.

SUSPENSION Y-PULLS

With your body facing the anchor point of the suspension trainer, hold onto the handles with your palms facing the floor and your arms straight and extended out in front of your shoulders (see figure *a*). Lean back with your body in a straight line from head to toe. Without bending your elbows, open your arms out diagonally to form a *Y* (see figure *b*). At the top of each rep, your body will end up being even with your arms. Slowly reverse the motion and lower yourself to the starting position to complete 1 rep. To increase the difficulty, start the exercise from a more severe backward lean, which brings your body closer to the floor.

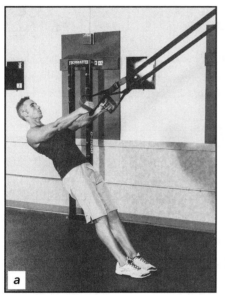
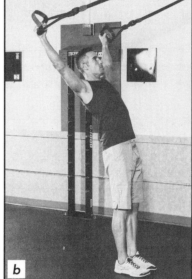

ONE-ARM BAND ROW

Stand tall, facing a band that's attached at roughly chest height to a stable structure or inside a doorjamb (many resistance bands come with an attachment for this). Hold both handles in your left hand and stand in a split stance with your left foot behind your right (see figure *a*). Pull the band toward your body (see figure *b*) and slowly let your arm straighten again without allowing your torso or hips to rotate. Perform all reps on one side before switching arms and reversing your stance.

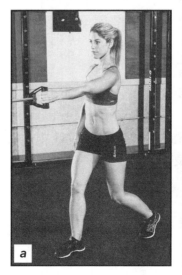
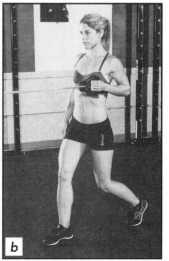

WIDE-GRIP BAND ROW

Stand tall with your feet hip-width apart and parallel to one another, facing a band that's attached at roughly shoulder height to a stable structure or inside a doorjamb (many resistance bands come with an attachment for this). Hold each handle with your palms down (see figure *a*). Pull the band toward you, keeping your elbows flared out from your body at a 90-degree angle (see

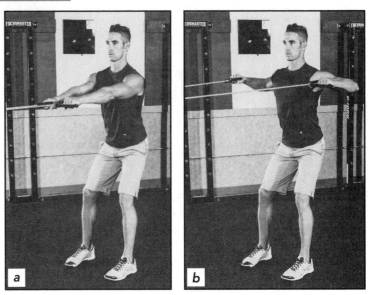

figure *b*). Slowly reverse the motion while keeping your spine straight and not allowing any extra body angles to occur. Be sure to keep your torso at an upright angle and pull your arms in a movement pattern that is parallel to the floor.

ALTERNATE-ARM BAND ROW

Stand tall facing a band that's attached at roughly chest height, holding one handle in each hand and standing in a split stance with your knees slightly bent (see figure *a*). As you pull the band toward your body with one arm (see figure *b*), let the other arm straighten without allowing your torso or hips to rotate. Alternate your arms in a quick motion.

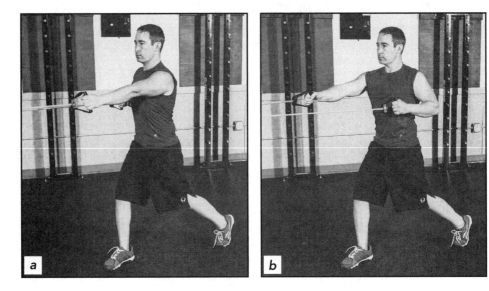

SPLIT SQUAT AND ONE-ARM BAND ROW

Stand tall facing a band that's attached at roughly chest height to a stable structure or inside a doorjamb (many resistance bands come with an attachment for this). Hold both handles in your left hand and stand in a split stance with your left foot behind your right. Lower your body toward the floor to perform a split squat (see figure *a*). As you come out of the squat, perform a one-arm row (see figure *b*). As you lower into your next squat, reverse the arm action of the row to complete 1 rep. Perform all reps on the same side before switching sides and reversing your stance.

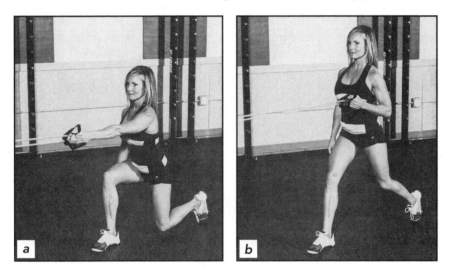

REVERSE LUNGE AND ONE-ARM BAND ROW

Stand tall with your feet hip-width apart, facing a band that's attached at chest height to a stable structure or inside a doorjamb (many resistance bands come with an attachment for this). Hold both handles in your left hand and step your left leg backward, dropping your knee lightly to the floor to perform a reverse lunge with both knees bent 90 degrees at the bottom of the lunge (see figure *a*). As you rise out of the lunge to bring your feet back to parallel, perform a band row by pulling your left arm into your side so that your wrist is by your ribs (see figure *b*). As you reverse the action of the row and extend your arm, simultaneously step backward again with your left leg.

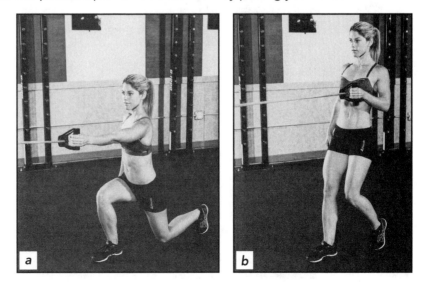

ONE-ARM BAND MOTORCYCLE ROW

Stand tall facing a band that's attached at roughly torso height to a stable structure or inside a doorjamb (many resistance bands come with an attachment for this). Hold both handles in your left hand and stand with your feet in a split stance with your left leg behind and your feet roughly shoulder-width apart. Hinge at your hips and lean your torso forward, keeping your knees bent 15 to 20 degrees (see figure a). Once your torso becomes parallel with the cable, perform a one-arm row by pulling your left arm into your side (see figure b). Allow your arm to straighten to complete 1 rep. Perform all reps on the same side before switching sides and reversing your stance.

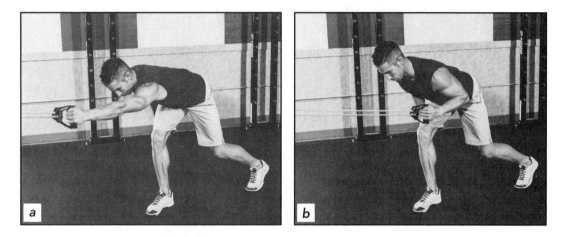

BAND SWIMMERS

Stand tall facing a band that's attached at roughly shoulder height to a stable structure or inside a doorjamb (many resistance bands come with an attachment for this). Hold one handle in each hand and stand with your feet in a parallel stance roughly shoulder-width apart (see figure a). With your arms straight, pull the band toward you, driving your thumbs toward your pockets and leaning forward by hinging at your hips (see figure b). At the bottom of each repetition, the band should be touching the tops of your shoulders and your arms and torso should be in the same line as the band. Reverse the motion, returning to the starting position with your arms straight out in front of you.

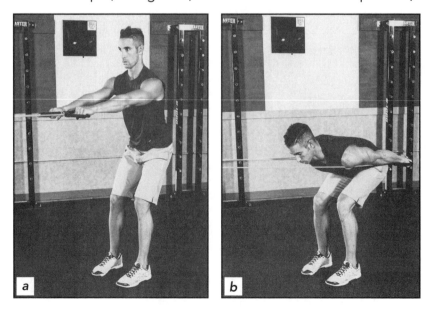

BAND BENT-OVER ROW

Stand tall facing a band that's attached at a low position (just above the ground) to a stable structure or inside a doorjamb (many resistance bands come with an attachment for this). Holding one handle in each hand, lean your torso at a 45-degree angle with your knees soft and your back straight (see figure *a*). Pull the band toward your body so that your wrists come by your ribs, ensuring that you squeeze your shoulder blades together every time you pull your arms in (see figure *b*). Reverse the motion by extending your arms back outward without allowing your lower back to round out or losing your stance.

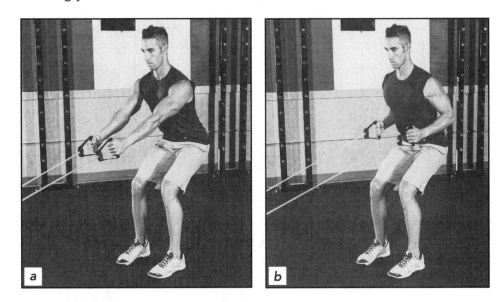

COMPOUND BAND ROW

Stand with your feet roughly shoulder-width apart and knees slightly bent, facing a band that is attached at midtorso to shoulder level to a stable structure or inside a doorjamb (many resistance bands come with an attachment for this). Hold the handles of the band in your right hand and hinge at your hips, with a slight bend at your knees and your arms extended above your head toward the anchor point (see figure *a*). Your arms should form a straight line between the band and your torso. Reverse this motion while simultaneously performing a row, finishing the row at the same time you return to standing upright (see figure *b*). Slowly reverse the motion, hinging at your hips and reaching out using good rhythm and coordination. You can also perform a one-arm version by holding both handles in one hand. Perform all the reps on one side before switching to the other side.

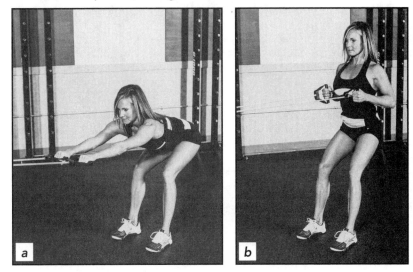

BAND LAT PULL-DOWN

Stand with your feet shoulder-width apart and face a resistance band that's attached at shoulder level to a stable structure or inside a doorjamb (many resistance bands come with an attachment for this purpose). Hold one handle of the band in each hand and bend over at your hips with a slight bend at your knees and arms extended above your head toward the anchor point of the band (see figure a). Your arms should be stretched out above your head, forming a straight line between the band, your arms, and your torso. Pull your arms into your sides the same as you would when using a lat pull-down machine so that your triceps come into contact with the sides of your body (see figure b). Slowly straighten your arms again to complete 1 rep. Be sure to keep your spine straight and do not round your lower back at any point in this exercise, and maintain a soft (20-degree) knee bend throughout.

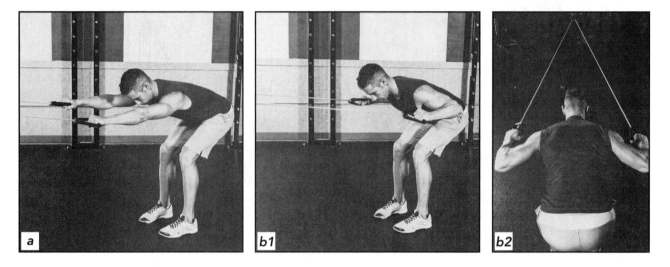

SUSPENSION BICEPS CURL

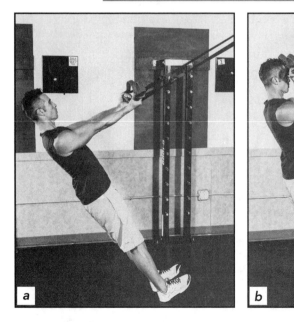

With your palms facing the ceiling and your body facing the anchor point, hold onto the handles and lean back with your body in a straight line from head to toe with your elbows straight and extended out in front of your shoulders (see figure a). Bending only at your elbows, perform a biceps curl and pull yourself up so that the handles touch your forehead (see figure b). Reverse the action to complete 1 rep.

Be sure to keep your body straight throughout the exercise. To increase the difficulty, start the exercise from a more severe backward lean which brings your body closer to the floor.

BALL BACK EXTENSION WITH ARM Y

Place your chest on the ball with your knees bent and your torso parallel to the floor with your arms hanging from your shoulders (see figure *a*). Raise your arms out to shoulder height, pointing your thumbs toward the sky (see figure *b*).

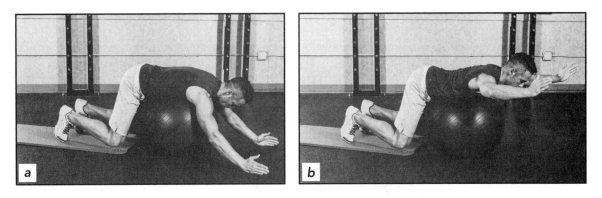

Body-Weight Abdominal Exercises

Although many of the exercises described thus far also work much of your core musculature, it's often the muscles on the backside along with the lateral torso muscles that have the most influence in those exercises. This is where the next exercises come in—they focus on the anterior abdominal muscles. Following is a list of creative exercises you can use to strengthen your abdominal muscles using only your body weight.

ARM WALK-OUT

From a kneeling position with your hands on the floor and your elbows straight (see figure *a*), walk your arms out in front of you as far as possible without allowing your lower back to extend beyond the starting position (see figure *b* and *c*). Reverse the motion, walking your hands back so your hands end up just in front of your shoulders.

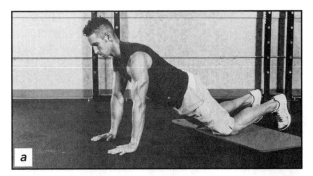

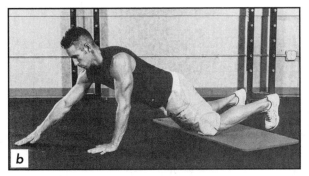

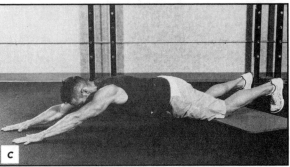

(continued)

(continued)

If you feel pressure in your lower back as you walk your hands out, you've gone too far beyond your strength threshold. Simply reduce your range of motion so you can perform the exercise in a pain-free manner. If bad wrists prevent you from doing this exercise, you can also perform roll-outs using a stability ball with your forearms on top of the ball, rolling it away from you and back underneath you.

BAND ANTIROTATION PRESS

Stand perpendicular to a band that's attached at shoulder height to a stable structure or inside a doorjamb (many resistance bands come with an attachment for this).

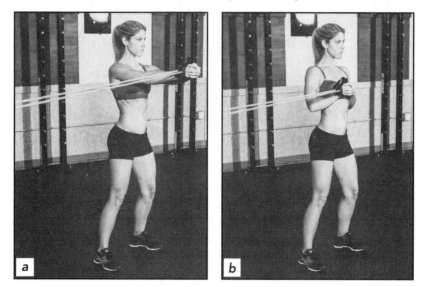

Hold both handles with both hands and reach your arms straight out in front of you at shoulder height without allowing your torso to rotate toward the band (see figure a). Then slowly reverse the action and bring your hands back into the center of your chest (see figure b). Be sure to stand tall and keep your feet shoulder-width apart. Perform all reps on one side before switching to the other side.

BAND TIGHT ROTATION

Stand with your feet shoulder-width apart with the handles of a resistance band on your right side at shoulder level; the band should be attached to a stable structure or inside a doorjamb (many resistance bands come with an attachment for this). Hold

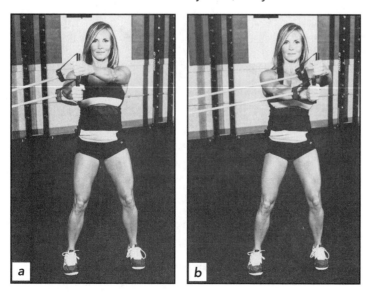

the handles on your right side with your elbows slightly bent (see figure a) and pull the handles across your body to the left until both arms are just outside your left shoulder (see figure b). Move your arms horizontally in the opposite direction (toward the origin of the cable) until they reach just outside your right shoulder. The range of motion in this exercise is small, roughly the same as the width of your shoulders. Be sure that you remain tall and do not allow your hips to rotate—they should remain perpendicular to origin of the bands. Perform all reps on one side before switching to the other side.

ONE-ARM PLANK

Begin in a push-up position with your hands and feet shoulder-width apart (see figure *a*). Lift one arm off the ground and place it on your chest without allowing your shoulders or hips to rotate or allowing your head or belly to sag toward the floor (see figure *b*). Pause for several seconds before switching hands. You can choose to perform this exercise from the elbows, but you should place a pad, pillow, or folded towel under your elbows for protection. To make this exercise more difficult, raise the arm you lifted out to the side instead of across your chest.

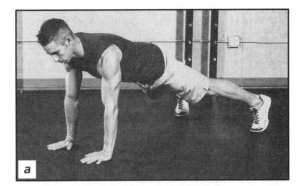
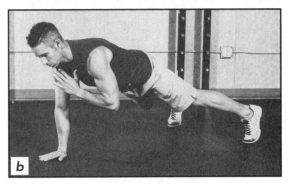

AB SNAIL

Sit on the floor with your legs outstretched and your hands supporting you just behind your hips (see figure *a*). Use your hands to push into the ground and raise

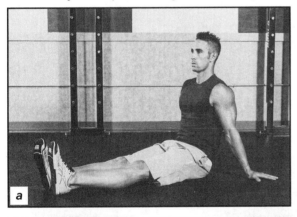

your hips (see figure *b*). Then pull your hips through your hands as far as possible and slowly lower them to the floor (see figure *c*). Place your hands behind you again and repeat, moving across the floor as you perform each repetition. Although this exercise can be performed almost anywhere, it's most convenient to do it on a surface that you can slide your feet across. As an aid you can place your heels on a paper plate.

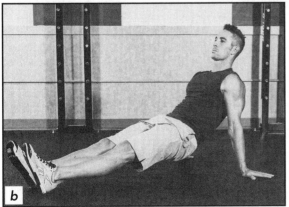
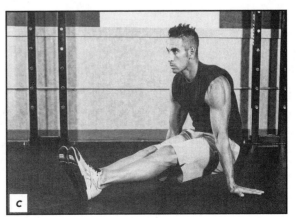

SUSPENSION AB FALL-OUT

Facing away from the anchor point of a suspension trainer, grab the handles and lean your weight forward in a push-up position (see figure *a*). Without bending your elbows, reach your arms above your head as if you were diving into a pool (see figure *b*). Pull your arms back in to complete 1 rep. Do not allow your hips to sag toward the floor. To increase the difficulty, start the exercise from a more severe forward lean, which brings your body closer to the floor.

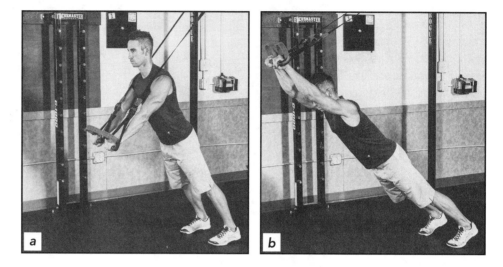

BALL ROLL-OUT

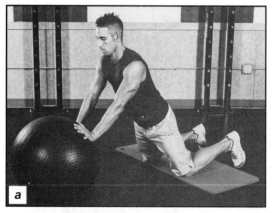

Kneel on the floor with your arms straight and your palms on a 55- to 65-centimeter stability ball with your knees and hands hip-width apart (see figure *a*). Drive the ball away from you by extending your arms overhead as if you were diving into a pool (see figure *b*). Push the ball out as far as you can without allowing your head or lower back to sag toward the floor (see figure *c*). Once you've gone as far as you can or your arms are completely up overhead in a straight line with your torso, reverse the motion and pull the ball back to the starting position where your hands are just above your head. To make this exercise easier, simply begin with your forearms resting on top of the ball, and perform the rest of the exercise as described.

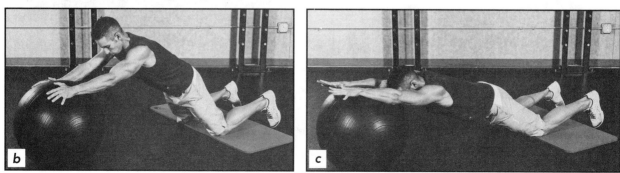

STABILITY-BALL STIR THE POT

Place both forearms on top of a fitness ball and assume a plank position with your body in a straight line and your feet shoulder-width apart (see figure a). Move your arms in small circles (see figure b and c). Alternate between clockwise and counter-clockwise circles without allowing your head or hips to sag toward the floor.

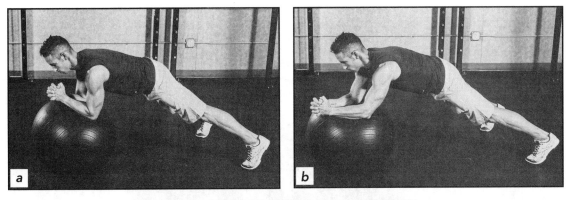

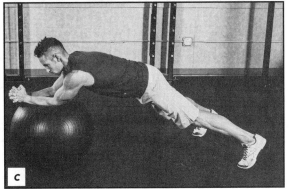

BALL KNEE TUCK

Assume a push-up position with your feet resting on top of a fitness ball that's between 55 and 65 centimeters in size (see figure a). Take your knees in toward your body as far as you possibly can without allowing your shoulders to move away from above your wrists where they started (see figure b). Reverse the motion so your body becomes straight again to complete 1 rep.

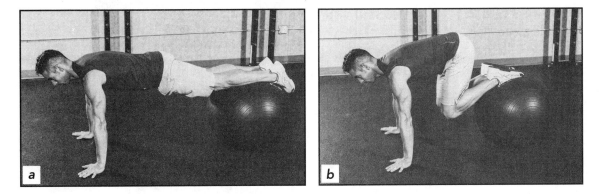

BALL PIKE

Assume a push-up position with your feet resting on top of a fitness ball that's between 55 and 65 centimeters in size (see figure a). Use your abs to raise your hips toward the sky, keeping your legs fairly straight. Raise your hips until just before they reach above your shoulders (see figure b). Slowly lower to the starting position with your body straight.

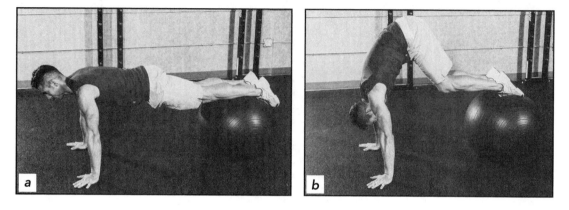

BALL PIKE ROLLBACK

This exercise combines the ball pike and the ball rollout into one comprehensive abdominal exercise. Hold yourself in a push-up position with your feet on a Swiss ball that's between 55-65 cm in size (to make the exercise easier, move the Swiss ball toward your belly button). With your body in a plank position (see figure a), keep your legs straight and push your hips towards the ceiling while keeping your back flat (see figure b). After straightening your hips and coming back to the start position, push your body backwards on the ball until your arms are fully extended in front of you and your legs are fully extended behind you (see figure c). Reverse the motion and repeat.

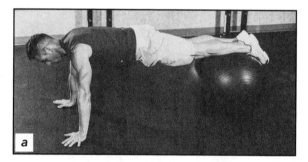

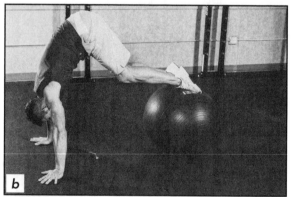

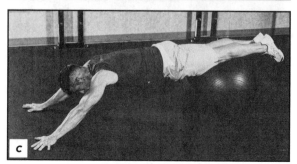

REVERSE CRUNCH

Lie supine on the floor with your knees bent and hips flexed into your belly (see figure a). With your elbows slightly bent, hold on to a dumbbell or medicine ball that's resting on the floor above your head. In a smooth controlled fashion perform a reverse crunch by rolling your lower back up off of the floor driving your knees toward your chin (see figure b). Slowly reverse this motion allowing your back to lower toward the floor one vertebrae at a time. Be sure to not use momentum and jerk your body in order to perform this exercise. Additionally, hold on to a dumbbell or medicine ball that is heavy enough to not allow you to lift it off of the ground while performing this exercise. Furthermore, your legs should not extend and your head should not lift off of the ground at any point during this exercise.

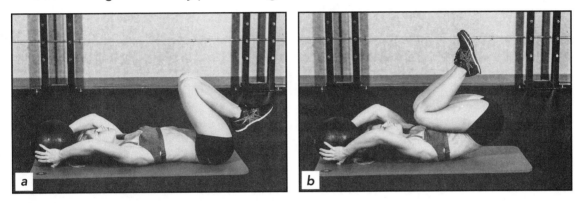

LEG LOWERING

Lie supine on the floor with your knees bent and hips flexed and fists on each side of your head pressing into the floor (see figure a). Slowly lower your legs toward the floor keeping your knees bent and pressure with your fist into the floor, without allowing your lower back to come off the floor (see figure b). Once your heels lightly touch the floor, reverse the motion bringing your knees back above your hips. To make this exercise more challenging simply extend your legs out further as you lower them towards the floor. Put simply, the further you straighten your legs, the harder the exercise. Just make sure that you never allow your lower back to lose contact with the floor at any point.

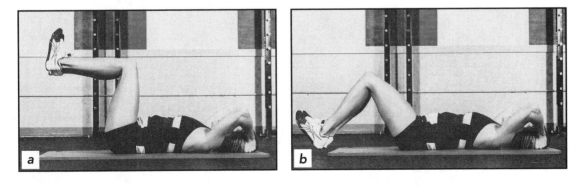

Body-Weight Combinations

As discussed in chapter 5, a strength training combination is a protocol that blends together multiple strength training movements to make one exercise. Following are metabolic strength training combinations that blend several of the previous body-weight exercises in a seamless and continuous fashion.

Burpee ▪ Frog Jump

This combination combines two dynamic movements into one total-body exercise. The two exercises flow together nicely because the end position of one sets you in the perfect position to start the other and vice versa. Following are the exercises for this combination.

1 BURPEE

With your feet slightly wider than shoulder-width apart, stand with your arm at your sides (see figure a). Bend your knees to squat down (see figure b) and jump your legs backward (see figure c) so you end up in a push-up position (see figure d). Make sure that your body forms one straight line and that you do not allow your hips to sag toward the floor. Jump your feet up (see figure e) and return to the tall standing position to complete the rep.

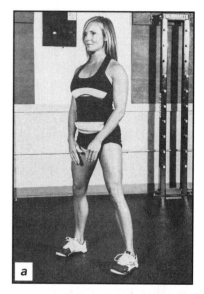

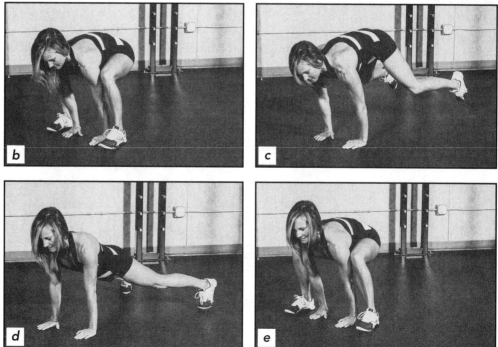

② FROG JUMP

With your knees bent roughly 20 degrees, hinge forward at your hips so that your back is parallel to the floor and your fingertips touch the ground in between your legs (see figure *f*). With a straight spine, explode into the air, straightening your body in midair (see figure *g*). Land as softly as possible and then drop back into the next burpee.

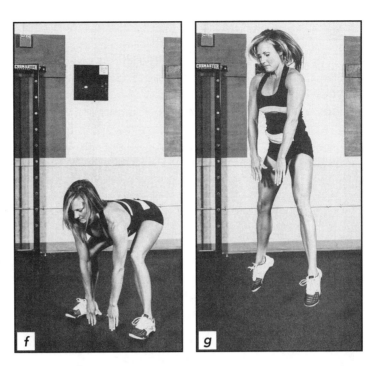

Squat Jump ▪ Down Burpee ▪ Break-Dancer Push-Up ▪ Up Burpee

This is a dynamic body-weight combination that has you changing your body's level by constantly getting up and down, which requires some coordination and athleticism. Perform one rep of each exercise before moving on to the next exercise. Then repeat the sequence from the beginning.

① SQUAT JUMP

Stand tall with your feet shoulder-width apart and your toes turned out slightly, about 10 degrees. Interlace your fingers behind your head with your elbows pointing out to the sides. Perform a squat by bending your knees and sitting back at your hips (see figure *a*). Go as low as you can possibly go without allowing your lower back to round out. As you squat down, be sure that you do not allow your heels to come off the ground or your knees to come together toward the midline. Your knees should track in the same direction as your toes. Quickly reverse the motion, jumping into the air as high as you can (see figure *b*). Land as lightly as possible back into the bottom of the squat position.

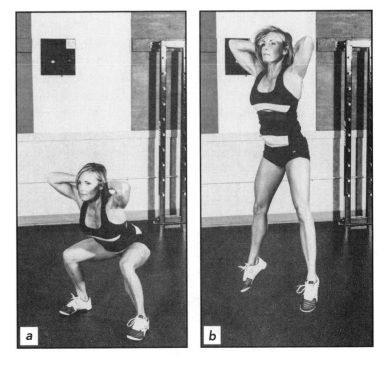

2 DOWN BURPEE

With your feet slightly wider than shoulder-width apart, stand with your arm at your sides (see figure c). Bend your knees to squat down (see figure d) and jump your legs backward (see figure e) so you end up in a push-up position (see figure f). Make sure that your body forms one straight line and that you do not allow your hips to sag toward the floor.

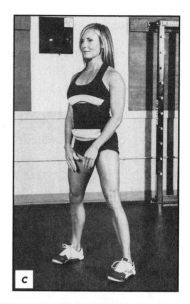

c

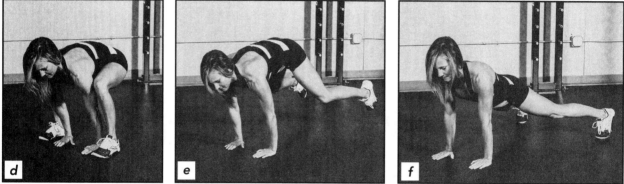

d   e   f

3 BREAK-DANCER PUSH-UP

Begin in a push-up position with your hands and feet shoulder-width apart. Perform a push-up (see figure g), and at the top of the repetition, rotate your entire body toward your left side, driving your right knee to your left elbow while keeping your left hand in front of your face (see figure h). Reverse this motion to perform another push-up and repeat this action on the opposite side, touching your left knee to your right elbow. Then, return to the starting push-up position.

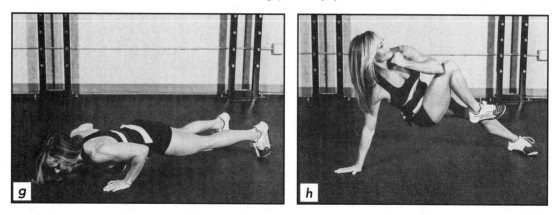

g   h

⁴ UP BURPEE

While in a push-up plank position (see figure *i*), jump your feet up so you are in a crouching position (see figure *j*). Then simply stand up tall.

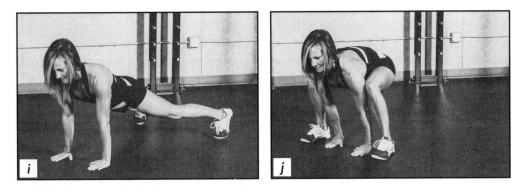

Frog Jump ▪ Down Burpee ▪ Push-Back Push-Up ▪ Up Burpee

This is a great combination for anyone who enjoys push-ups, because it combines two push-up variations back to back. It also intensely involves the hips and core muscles.

¹ FROG JUMP

With your knees bent roughly 20 degrees, hinge forward at your hips so that your back is parallel to the floor and your fingertips touch the ground in between your legs (see figure *a*). With a straight spine, explode into the air, straightening your body in midair (see figure *b*). Land as softly as possible in the starting position and move into the next exercise, down burpee.

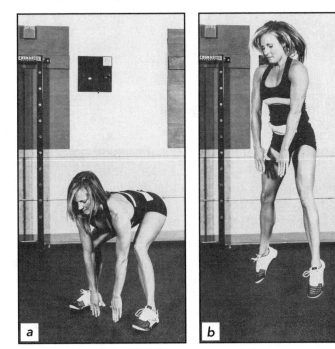

❷ DOWN BURPEE

With your feet slightly wider than shoulder-width apart, stand with your arm at your sides (see figure *c*). Bend your knees to squat down (see figure *d*) and jump your legs backward (see figure *e*) so you end up in a push-up position (see figure *f*). Make sure that your body forms one straight line and that you do not allow your hips to sag toward the floor.

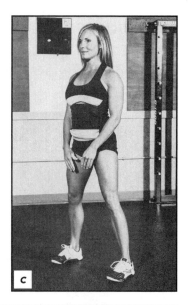

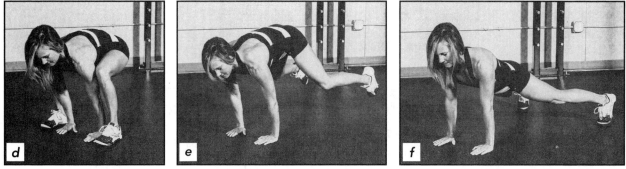

❸ PUSH-BACK PUSH-UP

Begin in a push-up position with your hands and feet shoulder-width apart (see figure *g*). Instead of pushing up out of the push-up in the traditional manner, soften your knees and push yourself backward toward your, feet keeping your hips as low as possible (see figure *h*). Reverse this motion and drop into the bottom of the push-up to complete 1 rep (see figure *i*).

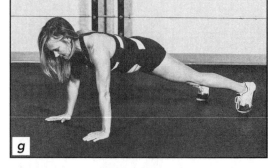

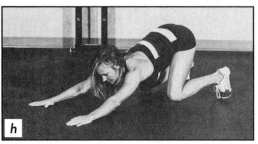

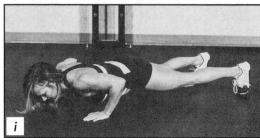

4 UP BURPEE

While in a push-up plank position (see figure *j*), jump your feet up so you are in a crouching position (see figure *k*). Then simply stand up tall.

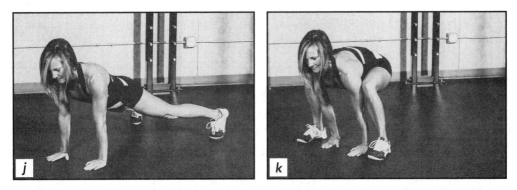

Body-Weight Complexes

As we covered in chapter 6, a strength training complex is a series of strength training exercises that are each performed for multiple reps using the same piece of equipment. In this case, the exercise equipment you'll be using is your own body weight. If you're looking to spice up some classic body-weight exercises, these metabolic complexes are just what the doctor ordered!

Squat Jump ▪ Push-Up ▪ Burpee ▪ Chin-Up or Pull-Up

Perform 4 squat jumps, then 3 push-ups, then 2 burpees, and finish with 1 chin-up or pull-up. After performing the reps provided for each exercise, repeat the sequence from the beginning.

1 SQUAT JUMP

Stand tall with your feet shoulder-width apart and your toes turned out slightly, about 10 degrees. Interlace your fingers behind your head with your elbows pointing out to the sides. Perform a squat by bending your knees and sitting back at your hips (see figure *a*). Go as low as you can possibly go without allowing your lower back to round out. As you squat down, be sure that you do not allow your heels to come off the ground or your knees to come together toward the midline. Your knees should track in the same direction as your toes. Quickly reverse the motion, jumping into the air as high as you can (see figure *b*). Land as lightly as possible back into the bottom of the squat position.

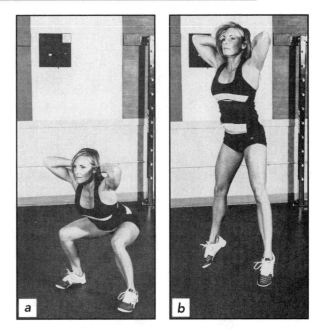

❷ PUSH-UP

With your hands on the floor just wider than shoulder-width apart and your elbows straight (see figure c), perform a push-up by lowering your body to the floor while keeping your elbows directly above your wrists the entire time (see figure d). Once your elbows have reached an angle just below 90 degrees, reverse the motion by pushing your body up so that your elbows are straight again.

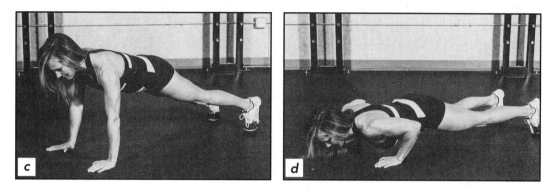

❸ BURPEE

With your feet slightly wider than shoulder-width apart, stand with your arm at your sides (see figure e). Bend your knees to squat down (see figure f) and jump your legs backward (see figure g) so you end up in a push-up position (see figure h). Make sure that your body forms one straight line and that you do not allow your hips to sag toward the floor. Jump your feet up (see figure i) and return to the tall standing position to complete the rep.

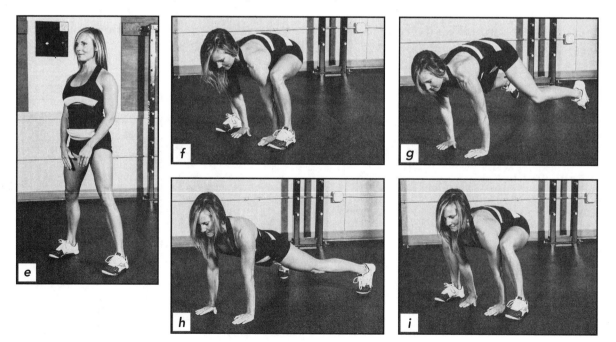

4 CHIN-UP OR PULL-UP

Hang from a bar with either a parallel underhand grip or wide grip (see figure *j*). Pull yourself up to the bar as powerfully as possible (see figure *k*) and then lower yourself in a slow and controlled manner, allowing no momentum or swinging.

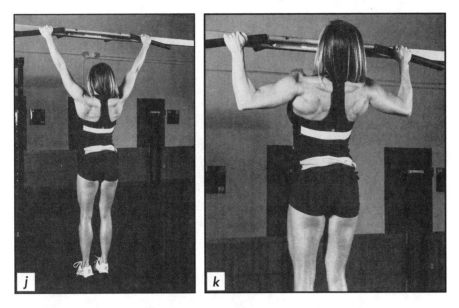

Overhead Reverse Lunge ▪ Down Burpee ▪ Break-Dancer Push-Up ▪ Up Burpee ▪ Frog Jump ▪ Chin-Up or Pull-Up

Perform 4 reverse lunges on each leg (8 total), then 3 break-dancer push-ups, then 2 frog jumps, and finish with 1 chin-up or pull-up. After performing the reps for each exercise, repeat the sequence from the beginning.

1 OVERHEAD REVERSE LUNGE

This is a great lunge option if you have limited training space because the mechanics are the same as in the walking lunge, except you don't move across the room and you step backward instead of forward. With your arms extended above your head and with your feet hip-width apart, step backward with one foot and drop your body so your knee lightly touches the floor (see figure *a*). Reverse the movement by coming out of the lunge and bringing your same foot forward so that you are back to your starting position (see figure *b*). Perform the same movement on the opposite leg.

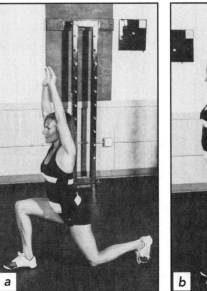
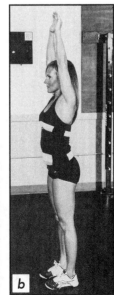

2 DOWN BURPEE

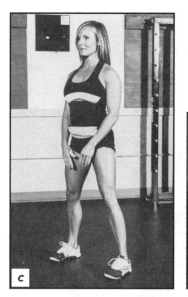

c

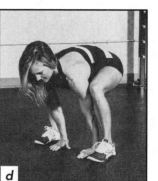

d

With your feet slightly wider than shoulder-width apart, stand with your arm at your sides (see figure *c*). Bend your knees to squat down (see figure *d*) and jump your legs backward (see figure *e*) so you end up in a push-up position (see figure *f*). Make sure that your body forms one straight line and that you do not allow your hips to sag toward the floor.

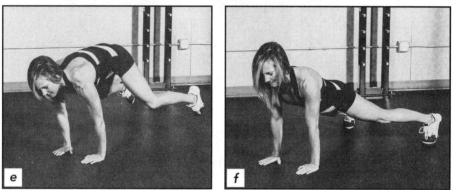

e

f

3 BREAK-DANCER PUSH-UP

Begin in a push-up position with your hands and feet shoulder-width apart. Perform a push-up (see figure *g*), and at the top of the repetition, rotate your entire body toward your left side, driving your right knee to your left elbow while keeping your left hand in front of your face (see figure *h*). Reverse this motion to perform another push-up and repeat this action on the opposite side, touching your left knee to your right elbow.

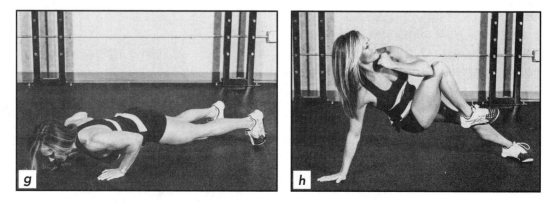

g

h

4 UP BURPEE

While in a push-up plank position (see figure *i*), jump your feet up so you are in a crouching position (see figure *j*). Then simply stand up tall.

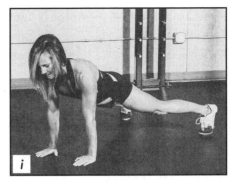

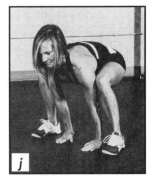

5 FROG JUMP

With your knees bent roughly 20 degrees, hinge forward at your hips so that your back is parallel to the floor and your fingertips touch the ground in between your legs (see figure *k*). With a straight spine, explode into the air, straightening your body in midair (see figure *l*). Land as softly as possible in the starting position and move on to the next exercise.

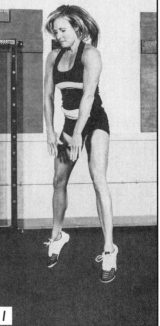

6 CHIN-UP OR PULL-UP

Hang from a bar with either a parallel underhand grip or wide grip (see figure *m*). Pull yourself up to the bar as powerfully as possible (see figure *n*) and then lower yourself in a slow and controlled manner, allowing no momentum or swinging.

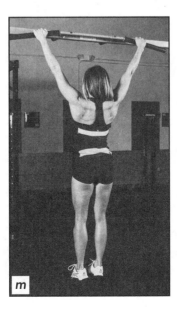

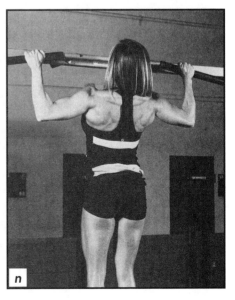

Two-Arm Compound Band Row ▪ Overhead Reverse Lunge ▪ Push-Back Push-Up ▪ Frog Jump

This complex uses a band to perform compound rows in place of chin-ups for times when you do not have access to a chin-up bar. Perform 5 compound rows, then 4 reverse lunges (8 total), then 3 push-back push-ups, and finish with 2 frog jumps. After performing the reps provided for exercise, repeat the sequence from the beginning.

1 TWO-ARM COMPOUND BAND ROW

Stand with your feet roughly shoulder-width apart and knees slightly bent, facing a band that is attached at midtorso to shoulder level to a stable structure or inside a doorjamb (many resistance bands come with an attachment for this). Hold one handle

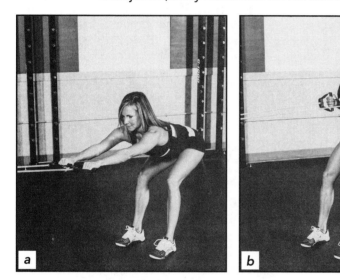

in each hand and hinge at your hips, reaching your arms above you toward the origin of the band (see figure a). Reverse this motion to stand up while simultaneously performing a row by pulling both arms into your chest, finishing the row at the same time you return to standing upright (see figure b). Slowly reverse the motion, hinging at your hips and reaching out using good rhythm and coordination.

2 OVERHEAD REVERSE LUNGE

This is a great lunge option if you have limited training space because the mechanics are the same as in the walking lunge, except you don't move across the room and you step backward instead of forward. With your arms extended above your head and with your feet hip-width apart (see figure c), step backward with one foot and drop your body so your knee lightly touches the floor (see figure d). Reverse the movement by coming out of the lunge and bringing your same foot forward so that you are back to your starting position. Perform the same movement on the opposite leg.

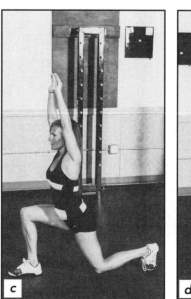
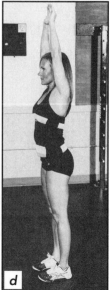

❸ PUSH-BACK PUSH-UP

Begin in a push-up position with your hands and feet shoulder-width apart (see figure e). Instead of pushing up out of the push-up in the traditional manner, soften your knees and push yourself backward toward your feet, keeping your hips as low as possible (see figure f). Reverse this motion and drop into the bottom of the push-up to complete 1 rep (see figure g).

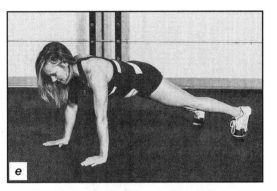

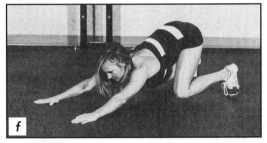

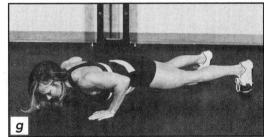

❹ FROG JUMP

With your knees bent roughly 20 degrees, hinge forward at your hips so that your back is parallel to the floor and your fingertips touch the ground in between your legs (see figure h). With a straight spine, explode into the air, straightening your body in midair (see figure i). Land as softly as possible in the starting position and repeat the jump.

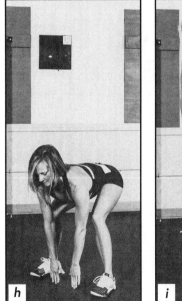

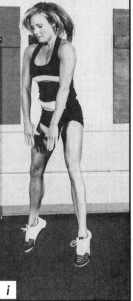

Arm Walk-Out ▪ Split-Squat Scissor Jump ▪ Break-Dancer Push-Up ▪ Up Burpee ▪ Frog Jump

Perform 4 arm walk-outs, then 3 split-squat scissor jumps (6 total), then 2 break-dancer push-ups, and finish with 1 up burpee into a frog jump.

1 ARM WALK-OUT

From a kneeling position with your hands on the floor and your elbows straight (see figure a), walk your arms out in front of you as far as possible without allowing your lower back to extend beyond the starting position (see figures b and c). Reverse the motion, walking your hands back so your hands end up just above your shoulders.

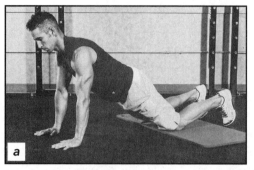

If you feel pressure in your lower back as you walk your hands out, you've gone too far beyond your strength threshold. Simply reduce your range of motion so you can perform the exercise in a pain-free manner. If bad wrists prevent you from doing this exercise, you can also perform roll-outs using a stability ball with your forearms on top of the ball, rolling it away from you and back underneath you.

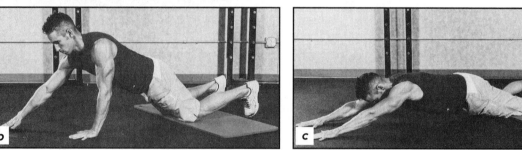

2 SPLIT-SQUAT SCISSOR JUMP

From a split stance with your fingers interlaced behind your head (see figure d), jump into the air, scissoring your legs (see figure e) so that you land with the opposite leg forward (see figure f). Jump into the air again, repeating this action. Be sure to land as quietly and as lightly as possible, using each landing to load the next jump.

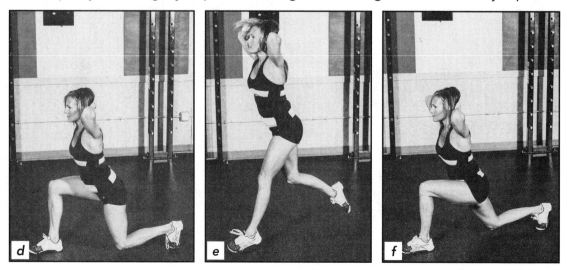

3 BREAK-DANCER PUSH-UP

Begin in a push-up position with your hands and feet shoulder-width apart. Perform a push-up (see figure *g*), and at the top of the repetition, rotate your entire body toward your left side, driving your right knee to your left elbow while keeping your left hand in front of your face (see figure *h*). Reverse this motion to perform another push-up and repeat this action on the opposite side, touching your left knee to your right elbow. Roll back to the push-up position.

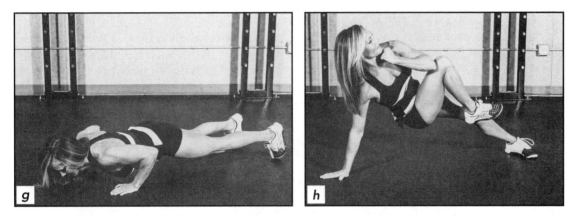

4 UP BURPEE

While in a push-up plank position (see figure *i*), jump your feet up so you are in a crouching position (see figure *j*). Then simply stand up tall.

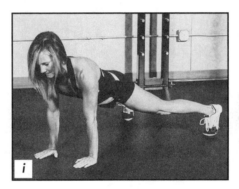
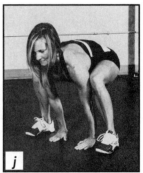

5 FROG JUMP

With your knees bent roughly 20 degrees, hinge forward at your hips so that your back is parallel to the floor and your fingertips touch the ground in between your legs (see figure *k*). With a straight spine, explode into the air, straightening your body in midair (see figure *l*). Land as softly as possible in the starting position and repeat the jump.

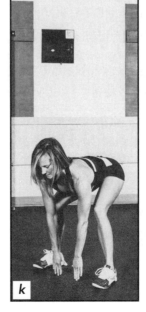
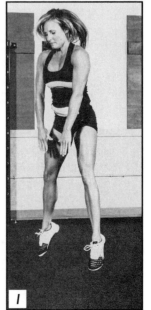

Lunge and Band Press ▪ Band Tight Rotation ▪ Split Squat and One-Arm Band Row

Using a set of heavy-duty resistance bands, perform 20 to 24 lunge and presses (alternating legs each lunge), then 20 to 24 tight rotations on each side, and finally 20 to 24 split squats and rows on each side.

1 LUNGE AND BAND PRESS

Face away from a band that's attached at roughly shoulder height to a stable structure or inside a doorjamb (many resistance bands come with an attachment for this). With your feet hip-width apart and in a parallel stance, hold a handle in each hand, with your elbows out to your sides and your forearms parallel to the floor (see figure a). Lunge forward while simultaneously performing a chest press with both arms, adding a slight lean forward to bring in your abdominal muscles (see figure b). Step back to the starting position, allowing your arms to come back as well. Repeat the press while lunging forward with the other leg.

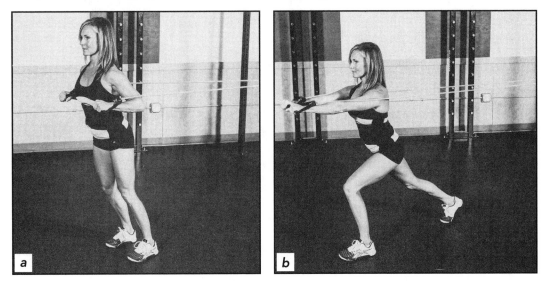

2 BAND TIGHT ROTATION

Stand with your feet shoulder-width apart with the handles of a resistance band on your right side at shoulder level; the band should be attached to a stable structure or inside a doorjamb (many resistance bands come with an attachment for this). Hold the handles on your right side with your elbows slightly bent (see figure c) and pull the handles across your body to the left until both arms are just outside your left shoulder (see figure d). Move your arms horizontally in the opposite direction (toward the origin of the cable) until they reach just outside your right shoulder. The range of motion in this exercise is small, roughly the same as the width of your shoulders. Be sure that you remain tall and do not allow your hips to rotate—they should remain perpendicular to origin of the bands. Perform all reps on the same side before switching sides.

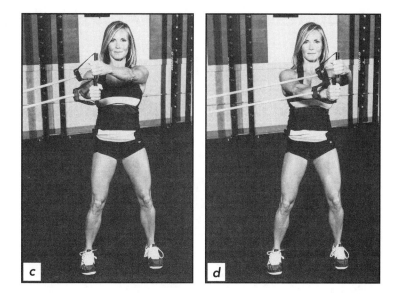

3 SPLIT SQUAT AND ONE-ARM BAND ROW

Stand tall facing a band that's attached at roughly chest height to a stable structure or inside a doorjamb (many resistance bands come with an attachment for this). Hold both handles in your left hand and stand in a split stance with your left foot behind your right (see figure e). Lower your body toward the floor to perform a split and as you come out of the squat, perform a one-arm row. As you lower into your next squat, reverse the arm action of the row to complete 1 rep (see figure f). Perform all reps on the same side before switching sides and reversing your stance.

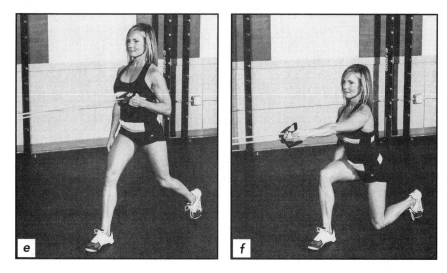

Reverse Lunge and One-Arm Band Row ▪ Band Tight Rotation ▪ One-Arm Band Press

This complex involves performing all repetitions using the same side. Perform 15 to 20 reverse lunge and rows pulling your with your left arm, then 15 to 20 tight rotations from right to left, and finish with 15 to 20 one-arm band presses with your left arm. Then repeat the complex using your right side.

1 REVERSE LUNGE AND ONE-ARM BAND ROW

Stand tall with your feet hip-width apart, facing a band that's attached at chest height to a stable structure or inside a doorjamb (many resistance bands come with an attachment for this). Hold one handle in each hand and step your left leg backward, dropping your knee lightly to the floor to perform a reverse lunge with both knees bent 90 degrees at the bottom of the lunge (see figure *a*). As you rise out of the lunge to bring your feet back to parallel, perform a band row by pulling your arm into your chest so that your wrist is up on the side of your ribs (see figure *b*). As you reverse the action of the row and extend your arm, simultaneously step backward with your left leg to perform a reverse lunge. Return to the parallel stance while performing the row again.

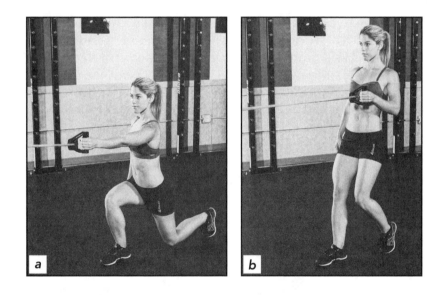

2 BAND TIGHT ROTATION

Stand with your feet shoulder-width apart with the handles of a resistance band on your right side at shoulder level; the band should be attached to a stable structure or inside a doorjamb (many resistance bands come with an attachment for this). Hold the handles on your right side with your elbows slightly bent (see figure c) and pull the handles across your body to the left until both arms are just outside your left shoulder (see figure d). Move your arms horizontally in the opposite direction (toward the origin of the cable) until they reach just outside your right shoulder. The range of motion in this exercise is small, roughly the same as the width of your shoulders. Be sure that you remain tall and do not allow your hips to rotate—they should remain perpendicular to origin of the bands.

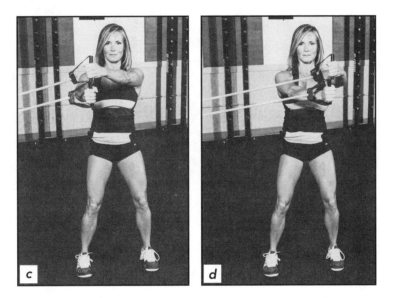

❸ ONE-ARM BAND PRESS

Face away from a band that's attached at roughly shoulder height to a stable structure or inside a doorjamb (many resistance bands come with an attachment for this). Stand in a split stance with your right leg in front and hold both handles of the band in your left hand (see figure e). Without allowing your torso to rotate, drive your arm straight out in front of you (see figure f). Slowly bring your arm back to complete 1 rep.

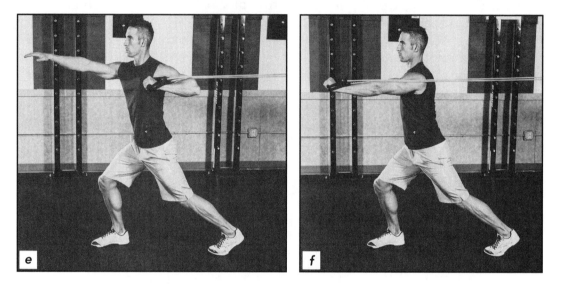

The take-away saying for this chapter is "No gym, no weights, no problem." You now have a multitude of new, fun, and challenging body-weight exercises all guaranteed to develop a rock-solid core, strong upper body, powerful legs and glutes, and lean body that won't quit. Wait until you see how some of these body-weight protocols have been put together in the workout programs provided in chapter 9. With those programs you'll see how to develop a world-class workout of metabolic strength training for fat loss at a moment's notice—wherever you are!

Warm-Ups and Cool-Downs for Fat Loss

This chapter covers the warm-up techniques and cool-down concepts you should use to bookend your metabolic strength training workouts. Although the title of this chapter is Warm-Ups and Cool-Downs for Fat Loss, just tacking on the phrase *fat loss* in no way gives these techniques special powers to burn body fat. These warm-up and cool-down applications are not in and of themselves an effective method for helping your body lose fat and maintain muscle. Rather, they are techniques that can enhance the productivity of your metabolic strength training efforts and offer some unique movement and health benefits that can make your training sessions more comprehensive.

WARM-UPS

Because your workout is dynamic, your warm-up must prepare your body for what's to follow by doing dynamic movements at a lesser intensity. Although static stretching may feel good and jogging may get your heart rate up, these methods don't prepare your brain or body for all the demands these workouts throw at you.

A dynamic warm-up is a transition stage from normal activity to more athletic activity. During this transition, you spend time doing some low-intensity strength training to activate some of the important muscles of your core (glutes, mid-back, and abdominal muscles), which often don't get used throughout day while sitting at home or at work. You also perform movements that increase overall mobility. These mobility movements help you do things like squat deeper, deadlift with a straighter back, and perform lifts with more comfort and less restriction. In addition, you perform a few athletic movement and coordination exercises, which not only get your heart rate up but also prepare your entire body for the more athletic, total-body workouts that follow.

The following warm-up sequences have been battle-tested to ensure that your brain and body are ready for anything! They work the whole body and can be done anywhere because they use little to no equipment and require little space. Additionally, each warm-up takes no more than 10 minutes. If you aren't willing to take 10 minutes to do something that helps you move and feel better and makes your workouts more productive, you may not be as serious about getting results as you think.

Dynamic Warm-Up

The exercises in the following dynamic warm-up will help you gain and maintain mobility and athleticism. This prepares you to focus on using the metabolic strength training workouts to maintain muscle while accelerating your metabolism to burn off that unwanted body fat.

Perform the following four exercises back to back in circuit fashion. Repeat the circuit for 2 to 3 rounds, resting no more than 30 seconds between rounds.

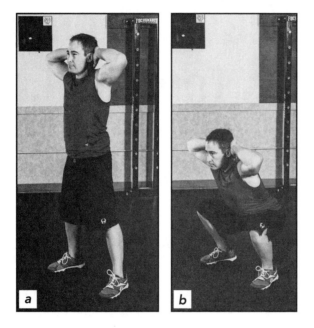

1 PRISONER SQUAT

Stand tall with your feet shoulder-width apart and your toes turned out slightly out, about 10 degrees (see figure *a*). Interlace your fingers behind your head with your elbows pointing out to the sides. Perform a squat by bending your knees and sitting back at your hips (see figure *b*). Go as low as you can possibly go without allowing your lower back to round out. Be sure that as you squat you do not allow your heels to come off the ground or your knees to come together toward the midline of your body. Your knees should track in the same direction as your toes. Repeat for 15 to 20 reps.

2 PUSH-UP

With your hands on the floor just wider than shoulder-width apart and your elbows straight (see figure *c*), perform a push-up by lowering your body to the floor while keeping your elbows directly above your wrists the entire time (see figure *d*). Once your elbows have reached an angle just below 90 degrees, reverse the motion by pushing your body up so that your elbows are straight again. Repeat for 6 to 12 reps.

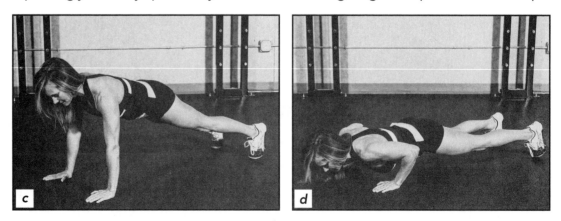

❸ T-ROLL

Assume a plank position with your wrists underneath your shoulders and your feet shoulder-width apart (see figure *e*). Rotate your entire body, moving your hips and shoulder at the same rate, reaching your top arm toward the sky (see figure *f*). Roll back to the starting position and repeat on the other side. Perform 6 to 8 reps on each side.

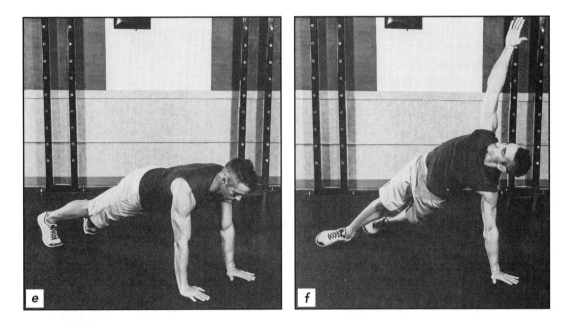

❹ ANTERIOR-REACHING LUNGE

Stand tall with your feet together (see figure *g*). Step forward, keeping your back leg straight and your front knee slightly bent. As you step forward, lean your torso forward, reaching your arms in front of you at waist height while keeping your back straight (see figure *h*). Step back to the starting position and repeat with the other leg. Perform 6 to 8 reps on each side.

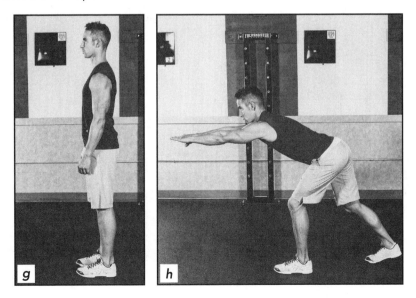

After you've completed 2 to 3 rounds of the four exercises just described, perform the following three exercises back to back in a circuit fashion and repeat for 1 to 2 rounds, resting no more than 30 seconds between rounds.

1 FROG JUMP

With your knees bent roughly 20 degrees, hinge forward at your hips so that your back is parallel to the floor and your fingertips touch the ground in between your legs (see figure *a*). With a straight spine, explode into the air, straightening your body in midair (see figure *b*). Land as softly as possible in the starting position and repeat the jump. Repeat for 3 to 5 reps on each side.

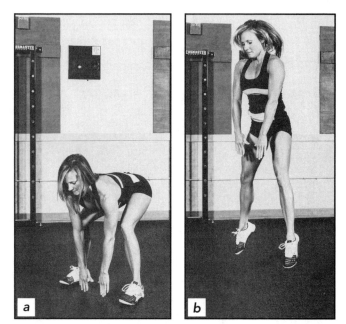

2 REVERSE LUNGE WITH OVERHEAD REACH

Stand tall with your feet together (see figure *c*). Step backward with one leg, dropping into a lunge position while simultaneously reaching both arms overhead and slightly leaning your torso backward (see figure *d*). Return to the standing position with your feet together and repeat by stepping back with the other leg. Repeat for 3 to 5 reps.

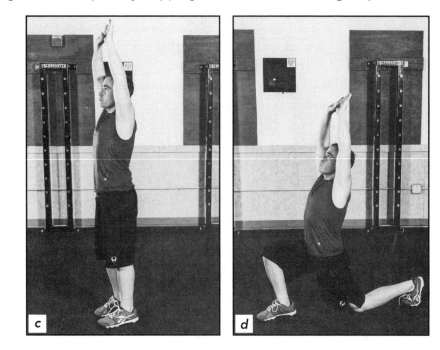

3 ROTATIONAL ARM SWING

Stand tall and reach your arms straight out in front of your shoulders (see figure e). Quickly rotate your torso to one side, driving both your hips and your arm behinds you (see figure f). Return to the starting position and repeat the same motion to the other side. Keep the motion fast and dynamic. Perform 5 to 8 reps on each side.

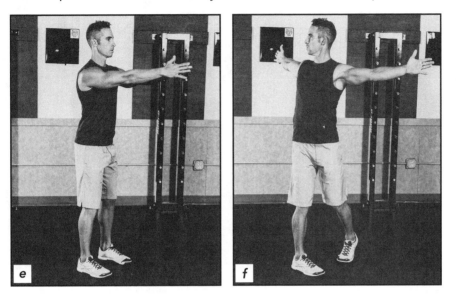

Stability-Ball Warm-Up

This is a great warm-up sequence for someone who wants to focus on the core musculature, which, as covered earlier in this book, includes all of your torso muscles, not just your abs. Not only is this warm-up sequence a great way to activate your entire core musculature, but it's also easy to memorize and offers a smooth transition from one exercise to the next.

A 55- to 65-centimeter stability ball is used for this warm-up. Perform the following four exercises back to back in a circuit fashion and repeat for 2 to 3 rounds, resting no more than 30 seconds between rounds.

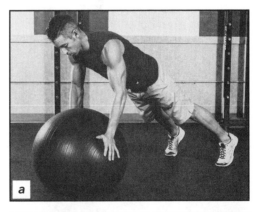

1 HANDS-ON-BALL PUSH-UP

Assume a plank position with your hands on a stability ball and your fingers pointing down toward the floor (see figure a). Lower your body and perform push-ups, keeping your back and neck straight throughout (see figure b). Repeat for 5 to 10 reps.

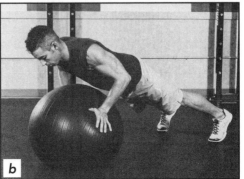

2 BALL BACK EXTENSION WITH ARM Y

Place your chest on the ball with your knees bent and your torso parallel to the floor with your arms hanging from your shoulders (see figure c). Raise your arms out to shoulder height, pointing your thumbs toward the sky (see figure d). Repeat for 10 to 15 reps.

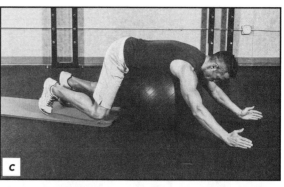

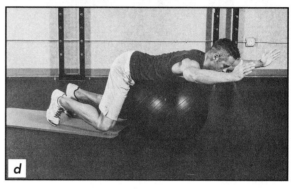

3 BALL KNEE TUCK

Assume a plank position with your hands on the floor and your shins resting on top of a stability ball (see figure e). Pull your legs into your body (see figure f) and bring them back out with good control. Repeat for 10 to 15 reps.

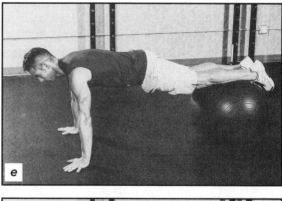

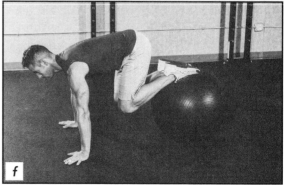

4 BALL HIP LIFT AND LEG CURL

Lie supine with your back on the floor and your heels resting on top of a stability ball (see figure g). Lift your hips up as you simultaneously bend your knees and pull the ball toward your body (see figure h and i. Slowly reverse the motion. Repeat for 10 to 15 reps.

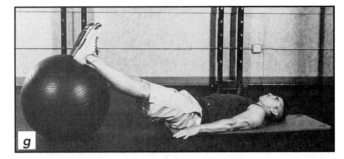

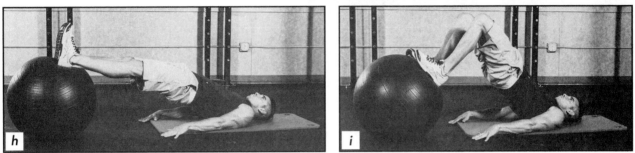

After you've completed 2 to 3 rounds of the four exercises just described, perform the following three exercises back to back in a circuit fashion and repeat for 1 to 2 rounds, resting no more than 30 seconds between rounds.

1 LATERAL LUNGE WITH SIDE ARM REACH

Stand with your arms by your sides (see figure a). Step to one side and lower into a side lunge while reaching overhead with far arm toward the side you stepped (see figure b). Your other hand should be by lunging foot. Step back to the middle and repeat on the other side. Repeat for 3 to 5 reps on each side.

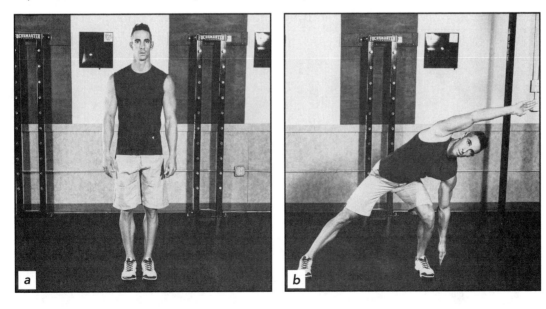

2 JUMPING JACK

Stand with your feet together and your hands at your sides (see figure c). As you raise your arms above your head, jump up just enough to spread your feet wide (see figure d). Without pausing, quickly reverse the movement. Repeat for 15 to 20 reps.

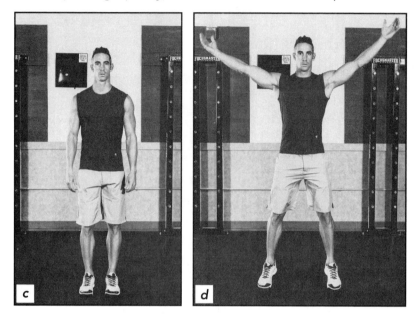

3 CROSSOVER JACK

Stand with your feet more than hip-width apart and your arms straight out to your sides at shoulder level (see figure e). Simultaneously cross your arms in front of your chest and jump up just enough to cross one leg in front of the other (see figure f). Without pausing, quickly reverse the motion and return to the starting position. Repeat, crossing your other leg in front and crossing your opposite arm on top. Repeat for 15 to 20 reps.

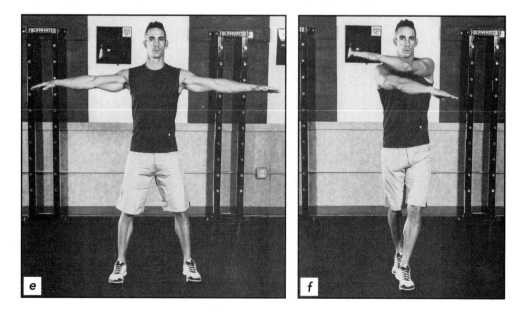

Resistance-Band Warm-Up

Similar to the stability-ball warm-up, this band warm-up is easy to memorize because it offers a smooth transition from exercise to exercise. Plus, it gets a lot done in a little time because it allows you to warm up your entire body by covering each of the basic movement patterns from the standing position.

A medium-load band is used for this warm-up. The band should be light enough to allow you to successfully complete the indicated reps with good control while creating enough resistance to offer an effective warm-up.

Perform the following four exercises back to back in a circuit fashion and repeat for 2 to 3 rounds, resting no more than 30 seconds between rounds.

1 ALTERNATING BAND ROW

Stand in a split stance facing where the band is anchored with your knees slightly bent and a handle in each hand (see figure *a*). Row one arm at a time in an alternating, cyclic action (see figure *b*). Keep a fast but controlled pace. Repeat for 20-30 total reps on each stance (i.e. 20-30 reps with your right leg forward and another 20-30 total reps with your left leg forward).

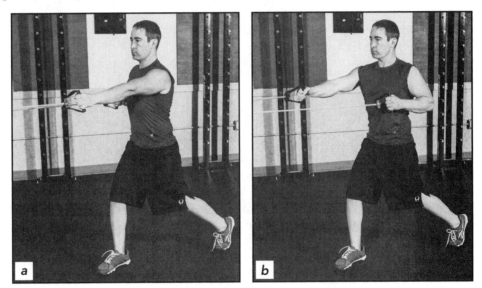

2 BAND TIGHT ROTATION

Stand with your feet shoulder-width apart with the handles of a resistance band on your right side at shoulder level; the band should be attached to a stable structure or inside a doorjamb (many resistance bands come with an attachment for this). Hold the handles on your right side with your elbows slightly bent (see figure *c*) and pull the handles across your body to the left until both arms are just outside your left shoulder (see figure *d*).

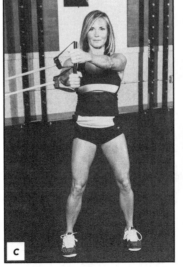
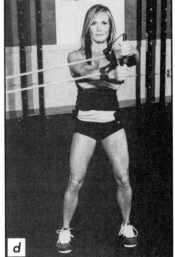

(continued)

(continued)

Move your arms horizontally in the opposite direction (toward the origin of the cable) until they reach just outside your right shoulder. The range of motion in this exercise is small, roughly the same as the width of your shoulders. Be sure that you remain tall and do not allow your hips to rotate—they should remain perpendicular to origin of the bands. Repeat for 10 to 15 reps on each side.

❸ LUNGE AND BAND PRESS

Facing away from where the band is anchored (see figure *e*), lunge forward with one leg while simultaneously performing a chest press with both arms (see figure *f*). Reverse the motion and step forward with the other leg while performing another chest press. Repeat in an alternating fashion. Repeat for 20 to 24 total reps.

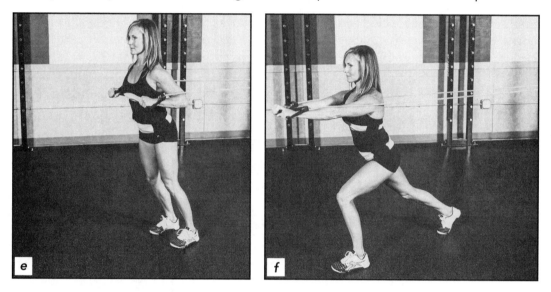

❹ PRISONER SQUAT

Stand tall with your feet shoulder-width apart and your toes turned out slightly out, about 10 degrees. Interlace your fingers behind your head with your elbows point-

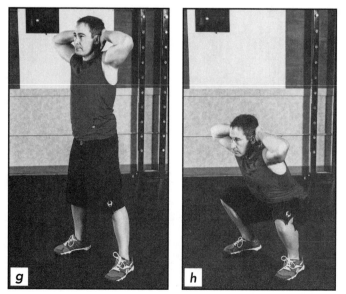

ing out to the sides (see figure *g*). Perform a squat by bending your knees and sitting back at your hips (see figure *h*). Go as low as you can possibly go without allowing your lower back to round out. Be sure that as you squat you do not allow your heels to come off the ground or your knees to come together toward the midline of your body. Your knees should track in the same direction as your toes. Repeat for 15 to 20 reps.

After you've completed 2 to 3 rounds of the four exercises just described, perform the following three exercises back to back in a circuit fashion and repeat for 1 to 2 rounds, resting no more than 30 seconds between rounds.

1 ARM CROSSOVER

Lie on your left side with your knees bent 90 degrees and straighten both arms in front of you, palms facing each other (see figure a). Keeping your left arm and both legs in position, rotate your torso to the right as far as you can until your right hand and upper back are flat on the floor (see figures b and c). Hold for 2 seconds and then return to the starting position. Repeat for 5 to 10 reps on each side.

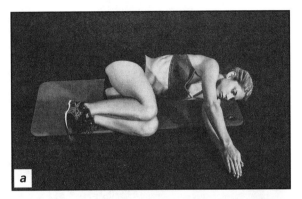

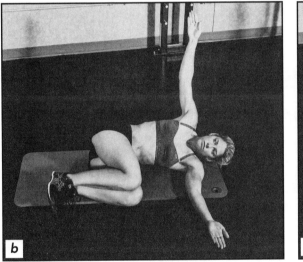

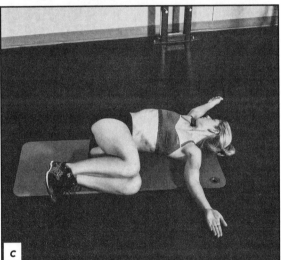

2 YOGA-PLEX

Begin in a push-up position and drive your hips backward and toward the sky so your body forms a triangle with your hips at the highest point (see figure d and e); this position is called *downward dog* in yoga. From this position your palms should be flat on the floor and you should be subtly pushing your heels toward the floor. Do not attempt to force your heels down to the floor; simply maintain a position that gives you a mild stretch in your calves and potentially your hamstrings. Slowly bring your left foot between your hands (see figure f) and rotate your torso to the left as you reach your left arm toward the ceiling (see figure g). Reverse back to the downward dog position. Repeat on the other side. Repeat for 3 to 5 reps on each side.

(continued)

(continued)

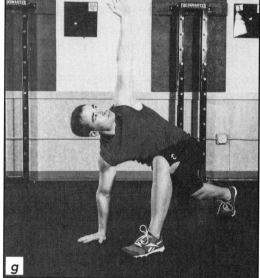

3 POGO HOPS

Stand tall with your feet under your hips, your elbows bent, and your hands pointing toward the sky (see figure *h*). As fast as possible, hop up and down in place, keeping your knees soft and using your arms to help drive each hop (see figure *i*). Repeat for 15 to 20 reps.

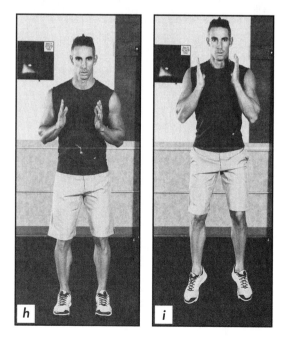

COOL-DOWN

Whereas a dynamic warm-up is a transition stage from normal activity to more athletic activity, a cool-down is just the opposite—it's a transition stage from more intense athletic activity to normal activity. Many exercisers simply like to do some light cardiorespiratory exercise 10 to 20 minutes as a cool-down, and that's perfectly okay. However, for many people this may not be sufficient to help them feel more relaxed and less tight after intense strength training such as the workouts featured in the following chapter.

One of the methods I recommend is self-massage using a foam roller, a rubber medicine ball, or a tennis ball (for smaller, more targeted areas). Self-massage techniques seem to create neuromuscular relaxation in the areas you are massaging, which can help the areas that are related to the ones you are massaging also relax because your body is an interconnected unit.

Regardless of the reasons why self-massage helps to increase range of motion and makes people feel better afterward, there is little argument that techniques such as those featured here can help you feel better, which is exactly why I recommend them.

Before we list the body areas where you can use self-massage, there are a few guidelines to go over:

- Roll the length of the muscle group you're massaging (up and down) 15 to 20 times or if you prefer to go for time, roll each area for 30 to 40 seconds.
- Start by placing the ball or roller in the middle of the area you're going to massage and work out from there.
- Beginning from the middle, roll the entire length of the muscle.
- Feeling tenderness (mild discomfort) is okay, but avoid painful spots.
- Only apply as much pressure as allows you to remain relaxed and maintain a normal breathing rate.
- Do not roll on injured or inflamed areas (such areas suffering from tendonitis).

Following is a description of how to use self-massage on various body areas.

Feet

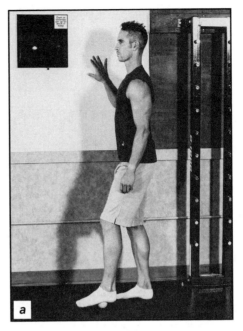

Place most of your weight on one leg while you roll a tennis ball up and down the length of the bottom of your other foot. It's okay to hold on to something for added balance if needed. See figure *a* for an example.

Calves

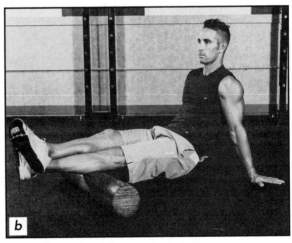

Sit with your legs outstretched and your right leg crossed over your left leg. With a foam roller underneath the center of your left calf, slightly lift your hips off the ground and use your arms to move your body over the roller and your top (right) leg to create some overpressure. Finish all rolls on one calf before switching to the other. See figure *b* for an example.

Mid-Back

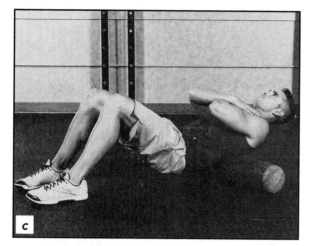

Lie supine on a foam roller so that it is positioned underneath your mid-back area. Cross your arms in front of your chest. With your hips off the ground, use your legs to move the roller up and down your mid-back (thoracic spine) region. See figure *c* for an example.

Quadriceps

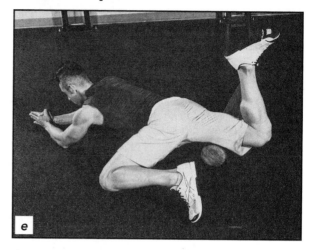

Assume a prone position on your elbows with your right thigh resting on top of the roller and your left knee bent away from your body. Use your arms to move your right thigh up and down the roller. Perform all rolls on your right thigh before switching sides. See figure *e* for an example.

Lats

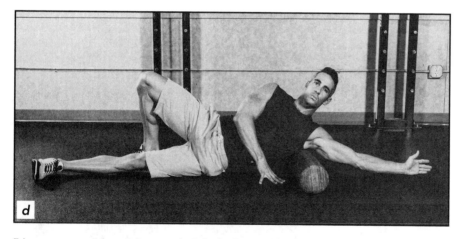

Lie on your side with your left latissimus dorsi resting on the roller and your left arm outstretched above you. Roll up and down the length of the muscle, and then repeat on the other side. See figure *d* for an example.

Glutes

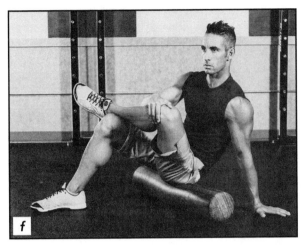

Sit on top of a foam roller or a medicine ball with it underneath your left glute. Cross your left leg over your right leg. Roll across your entire left gluteal region, making sure to cover the whole muscle area. Once you've finished all rolls on the left side, switch sides, cross your legs the opposite way, and roll on the right glute. See figure *f* for an example.

Pectorals and Biceps

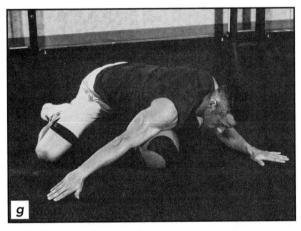

From a kneeling position with your legs spread, rest your right shoulder on top of a medicine ball with your right arm outstretched to your side and your left hand lightly supporting you on the floor. Roll the ball horizontally across your right arm from your biceps to your right pectoral area. After all rolls, switch to your left side and repeat. See figure *g* for an example.

If you have an area of your body that you think would feel better after self-massage that wasn't mentioned in this chapter, simply place a tennis ball on that spot and go to town. Just keep in mind the guidelines provided earlier, especially the one about avoiding inflamed areas, because rolling on them could increase irritation.

An extra benefit of the warm-up protocols and the self-massage (cool-down) methods provided in this chapter is that you can use them at any time throughout the day to help your body feel better and move better. If you are on the go and just want to get some brief exercise, performing a few rounds of one of the warm-up protocols provided in this chapter will certainly give you a light sweat and help reinvigorate you. The self-massage protocols are also something you can use throughout the day, whether at home or at the office, to help you feel more relaxed and loose. The self-massage techniques are the next best thing to getting a real massage, and you can use them at your convenience without the additional cost.

chapter

9

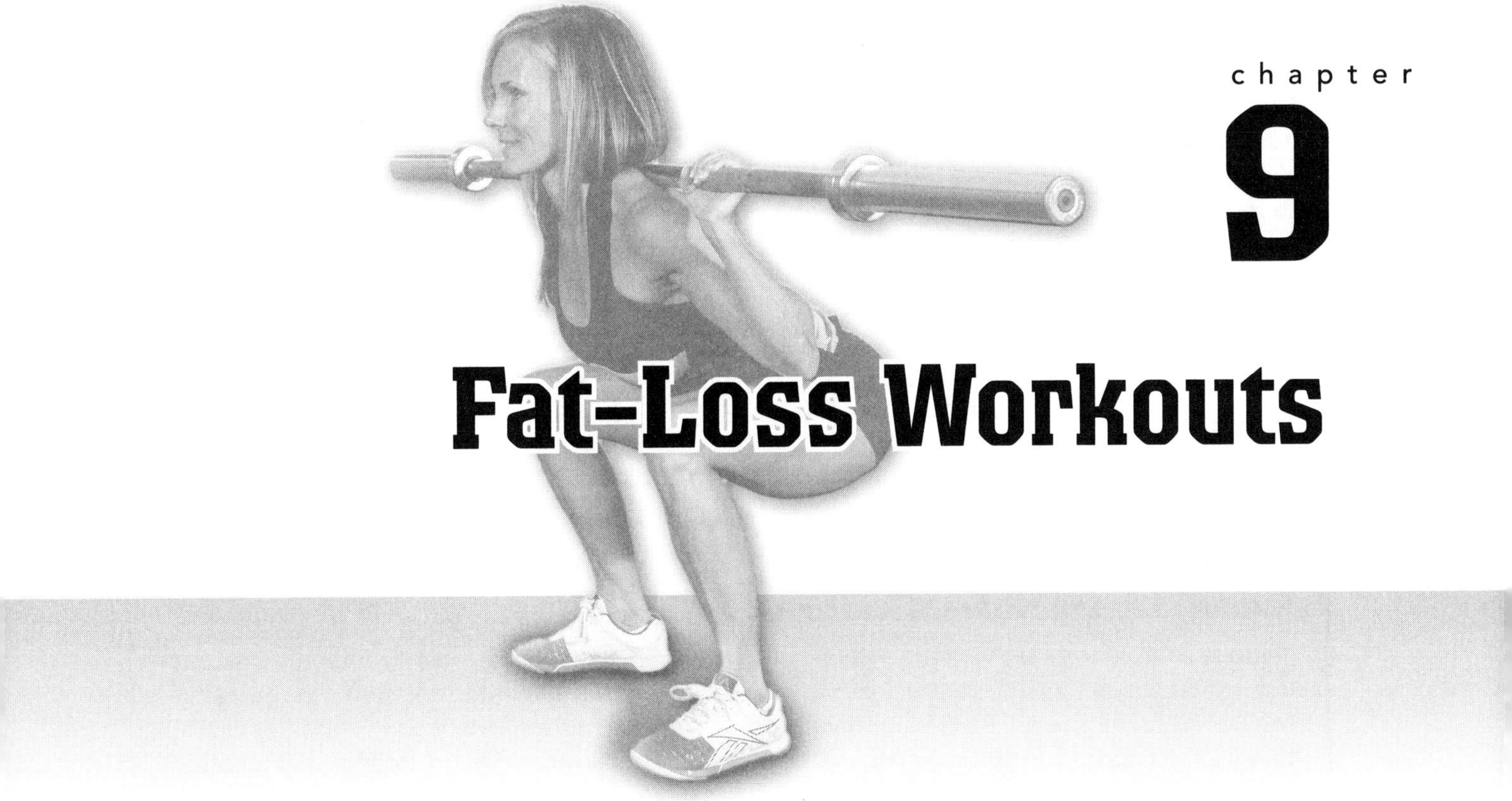

Fat-Loss Workouts

So far you've learned how to safely and effectively perform a wide variety of metabolic strength training exercises and protocols that you're surely excited to use. Now it's time to put all these great exercise concepts together into practical workout programs that, when combined with the nutritional habits discussed earlier, will help you improve your muscle and strength, getting you into great shape while you torch body fat.

The workout programs you'll find here are designed to help you make the most out of your time in the gym. Although the programs allow for ample rest time, you'll find they are exciting because they're fast paced and incorporate a variety of exercise protocols based on the three Cs. As you'll see, you have plenty of exercise programs to choose from to stay continually interested and challenged.

BREAK-IN WORKOUT PROGRAMS FOR BEGINNERS

If you're just starting out or it's been a while since you've done any strength training, I suggest that you perform the workout program in figure 9.1. Or, if you're more comfortable beginning your training at home, figure 9.2 provides another beginner program that uses only body-weight and band exercises.

For each of the beginner workouts, you will perform them 3 to 4 times per week for 2 weeks, but no more than 2 days in a row. You will perform *a* and *b* exercises as paired sets and complete all sets of *a* and *b* before moving on to the next paired set. Focus on the technique of each exercise, using deliberate control on each rep. Use a weight load that allows you to maintain good control. Additionally, do not take any of these sets to muscular failure, which means you should use a weight load that creates only mild muscle fatigue at the end of each set. Finally, before you begin your workout, you should perform a dynamic warm-up, and you should perform a cool-down at the end of the workout (see chapter 8).

Workout Rules and Recommendations

Your number one goal when using any fitness program is to avoid hurting yourself. And, the best way to ensure maximal safety when training is to focus on your lifting technique and use deliberate control in all of your exercises. Sure, these workout programs are intense, but doing an intense workout is not an excuse for poor technique. Here are a few key things to take note of before you start your workouts:

Substitute Equivalent Exercises

If you're unable to perform a given exercise using the techniques described earlier in the book, substitute an exercise equivalent that you're capable of doing in a controlled manner.

If you're using a workout program that features an exercise that gives you pain, simply substitute an equivalent exercise that you can perform without pain. We'll discuss this in greater detail in the next chapter.

Rest as Necessary

If you have to rest a bit longer than indicated in the workouts in order to complete the reps indicated with good control, please do so. This program emphasizes movement quality over quantity!

Use Appropriate Weight Loads

The weight loads shown in the photos that accompany each exercise are *not* an indication of the weight load you should use; it is purely for technique demonstration purposes. When performing exercises in a circuit, or when doing the finishing (isolation) exercises, which are often placed at the end of the each program, the weight load you use will be dictated by the repetitions provided. In that, if the workout program calls for 3 sets of 8-10 repetitions, you must use a weight load that allows you (on each set) to be challenged at 8 reps and unable to perform any more than 10 reps. In order to achieve this, when using the same weight load on each set, you may have to on the first set perform 10 reps, 9 reps on the second, and 8 reps on the third and final set in order to maintain the rep range provided while also accommodating for the accumulated fatigue that inevitably sets in as your workout progresses.

If you prefer to perform the same number of reps on each set, another option would be to use a weight that is roughly 5% lighter on each subsequent set. This approach accommodates for the 5-10% loss in strength that is commonly experienced on each set.[1]

Also, remember that when you are performing *combinations* or *complexes*, the weight load you use is dictated by the exercises or movement within it that you're weakest at. For example, let's say you're performing a complex that involves bent-over rows, Romanian deadlifts, hang cleans, and overhead push presses. You most certainly will be capable of lifting more weight in a Romanian deadlift than you will in the overhead push press.

Figure 9.1 Break-In Workout Program for Beginners

	Week 1	Week 2
1a. Goblet squat	1-2 sets x 6-8 reps	2-3 sets x 6-8 reps
1b. One-arm free-standing dumbbell row	1-2 sets x 8-10 reps (each side)	2-3 sets x 8-10 reps (each side)
2a. Barbell Romanian deadlift	1-2 sets x 8-10 reps	2-3 sets x 8-10 reps
2b. T-roll push-up	1-2 sets x 6-8 reps	2-3 sets x 6-8 reps
3a. Stability-ball leg curl	1-2 sets x 10-12 reps	2-3 sets x 10-12 reps
3b. One-arm overhead dumbbell press	1-2 sets x 6-8 reps (each side)	2-3 sets x 6-8 reps (each side)
4a. Chin-up or machine lat pull-down	1-2 sets x 8-10 reps	2-3 sets x 8-10 reps
4b. Dumbbell or prisoner reverse lunge	1-2 sets x 6-8 reps (each side)	2-3 sets x 6-8 reps (each side)
5. Cable or band tight rotation	1-2 sets x 10-12 reps (each side)	2-3 sets x 10-12 reps (each side)

Figure 9.2 Break-In At-Home Workout Program for Beginners

	Week 1	Week 2
1a. Prisoner squat	2 sets x 8-12 reps	3 sets x 8-12 reps
1b. One-arm compound band row	2 sets x 10-12 reps (each side)	3 sets x 10-12 reps (each side)
2a. Knee-tap squat	2 sets x 6-8 reps (each side)	3 sets x 6-8 reps (each side)
2b. Push-up	2 sets x 8-12 reps	3 sets x 8-12 reps
3a. Stability-ball leg curl	2 sets x 8-10 reps	3 sets x 8-10 reps
3b. One-arm band press	2 sets x 10-12 reps (each side)	3 sets x 10-12 reps (each side)
4a. Band lat pull-down	2 sets x 10-12 reps	3 sets x 10-12 reps
4b. Prisoner reverse lunge	2 sets x 4-6 reps (each side)	3 sets x 4-6 reps (each side)
5a. Band tight rotation	2 sets x 10-12 reps (each side)	3 sets x 10-12 reps (each side)
5b. Stability-ball knee tuck	2 sets x 8-10 reps	3 sets x 8-10 reps

MUSCLE-BASE WORKOUT PROGRAM

If you have been using strength training or if you've finished one of the 2-week break-in programs provided previously, you'll use the 4-week muscle-base training program to ensure your body is ready to perform the more intense workouts using the three Cs of metabolic strength training. After you've completed 4 weeks of the muscle-base training program shown in figures 9.3a and 9.3b, you're ready to use any of the sample workout programs that are provided later in this chapter.

The following program is based on two workouts: workout A and workout B. You'll perform this program 4 times per week, but no more than 2 days in a row. Although both workouts involve both the upper and lower body, each one focuses on different areas of the body, as follows:

- *Workout A:* quadriceps, lats, mid-back, abs, calves, biceps
- *Workout B:* hamstrings, glutes, chest, obliques, shoulders, triceps

Because this program is designed to maximize muscle growth along with connective tissue strength, it allows you to hit each muscle group with enough work volume to create a stimulus for growth while also allowing optimal recovery between workouts. In other words, while you're doing workout B, you are allowing all the muscles you hit in workout A to recover, but you are remaining active both days, which allows you to work out more often and thus increase your fitness level faster.

Figure 9.3*a*   Muscle-Base Workout Program A

	Week 1	Week 2	Week 3	Week 4
1a. Barbell front squat	2 sets x 6-8 reps	2 sets x 8-10 reps	3 sets x 6-8 reps	3 sets x 12, 10, 8 reps
1b. One-arm free-standing dumbbell row	2 sets x 8-10 reps (each side)	2 sets x 10-12 reps (each side)	3 sets x 8-10 reps (each side)	3 sets x 14, 12, 10 reps (each side)
2a. Dumbbell reverse lunge	2 sets x 6-8 reps	2 sets x 8-10 reps	3 sets x 6-8 reps	3 sets x 12, 10, 8 reps
2b. Chin-up or machine lat pull-down	2 sets x 6-8 reps	2 sets x 8-10 reps	3 sets x 6-8 reps	3 sets x 12, 10, 8 reps
3a. Dumbbell bench step-up (alternate legs)	2 sets x 6-8 reps (each side)	2 sets x 8-10 reps (each side)	3 sets x 6-8 reps (each side)	3 sets x 12, 10, 8 reps (each side)
3b. Dumbbell plank row	2 sets x 6-8 reps	2 sets x 8-10 reps	3 sets x 6-8 reps	3 sets x 12, 10, 8 reps
4a. Barbell calf raise	2 sets x 8-10 reps	2 sets x 10-12 reps	3 sets x 8-10 reps	3 sets x 15, 12, 10 reps
4b. Dumbbell biceps curl	2 sets x 6-8 reps (each side)	2 sets x 8-10 reps (each side)	3 sets x 6-8 reps (each side)	3 sets x 12, 10, 8 reps (each side)
5a. Ball roll-out	2 sets x 10-12 reps	2 sets x 12-14 reps	3 sets x 10-12 reps	3 sets x 12-14 reps
5b. Stability-ball knee tuck	2 sets x 8-10 reps	2 sets x 10-12 reps	3 sets x 8-10 reps	3 sets x 10-12 reps

Figure 9.3*b*   Muscle-Base Workout Program B

	Week 1	Week 2	Week 3	Week 4
1a. Romanian deadlift (with barbell)	2 sets x 6-8 reps	2 sets x 8-10 reps	3 sets x 6-8 reps	3 sets x 12, 10, 8 reps
1b. Box crossover push-up	2 sets x 4-6 reps (each side)	2 sets x 6-8 reps (each side)	3 sets x 4-6 reps (each side)	3 sets x 10, 8, 6 reps (each side)
2a. Horizontal hip extension	2 sets x 8-10 reps	2 sets x 10-12 reps	3 sets x 8-10 reps	3 sets x 12, 10, 8 reps
2b. One-arm overhead press (with dumbbell)	2 sets x 4-6 reps (each side)	2 sets x 6-8 reps (each side)	3 sets x 4-6 reps (each side)	3 sets x 10, 8, 6 reps (each side)
3a. One-leg hip thrust (pause 2 sec at top of rep)	2 sets x 6-8 reps (each side)	2 sets x 8-10 reps (each side)	3 sets x 6-8 reps (each side)	3 sets x 12, 10, 8 reps (each side)
3b. Chest press (with dumbbells)	2 sets x 6-8 reps	2 sets x 8-10 reps	3 sets x 6-8 reps	3 sets x 12, 10, 8 reps
4a. Side plank to dumbbell lateral raise	2 sets x 6-8 reps	2 sets x 8-10 reps	3 sets x 6-8 reps	3 sets x 12, 10, 8 reps
4b. Triceps dumbbell skull crusher	2 sets x 6-8 reps	2 sets x 8-10 reps (each side)	3 sets x 6-8 reps (each side)	3 sets x 12, 10, 8 reps (each side)
5a. Stability-ball leg curl	2 sets x 10-12 reps	2 sets x 12-14 reps	3 sets x 10-12 reps	3 sets x 12-14 reps
5b. Stability-ball stir the pot	2 sets x 15-20 sec	2 sets x 15-20 sec	3 sets x 15-20 sec	3 sets x 15-20 sec

METABOLIC STRENGTH TRAINING WORKOUT PROGRAMS

Now it's time for you to see how you can put exercise techniques together to form comprehensive workout programs. The following sample workouts involve each of the three Cs of metabolic strength training: complexes, circuits, and combinations. But before you get going with any of these programs, it's important that you know when and how often to use them each week. Here's what you need to know about using these metabolic strength training workouts.

Metabolic Strength Training Workouts

The following six workout programs in figures 9.4 through 9.15 are composed of two parts, workout A and workout B, that you alternate between. Each workout program is designed to be performed 4 days per week, but no more than 2 days in a row, for a duration of 4 weeks before changing to another program in order to keep your workout from getting stale and boring.

I've given you plug and play workout programs that can easily be adjusted to any training environment. It's okay and, in fact, I encourage you to substitute exercises in the following workout programs and replace them with similar exercises from the same category in order to accommodate your particular training environment. In other words, if there is a particular upper-body pushing exercise that you're unable to utilize or you don't have the ability to perform, insert a different upper-body pushing exercise in its place that better fits your training situation and ability.

It's important to note that these workout programs are provided to help you hit the ground running (in the right direction) by showing you how these metabolic strength training concepts and techniques can be put together in a variety of ways to develop comprehensive workout programs. So, don't just follow these workout programs, but also use them as templates to structure and develop you own endless variety of metabolic strength training workouts.

Figure 9.4 Metabolic Strength Training Program 1: Workout A

	Week 1	Week 2	Week 3	Week 4
Barbell combination	*8 min total (as fast as possible)*	*9 min total (as fast as possible)*	*10 min total (as fast as possible)*	*10 min total (as fast as possible) (use a heavier load than week 3)*
Bent-over row	1 rep	1 rep	1 rep	1 rep
Romanian deadlift	2 reps	2 reps	2 reps	2 reps
Hang clean	1 rep	1 rep	1 rep	1 rep
Overhead push press	1 rep	1 rep	1 rep	1 rep
	Rest 3-4 min.	Rest 3-4 min.	Rest 2-3 min.	Rest 2-3 min.
Big 4 circuit	*4-5 sets total*	*4-5 sets total*	*4-5 sets total*	*4-5 sets total*
Chin-up or lat pull-down (underhand grip)	6-8 reps	6-8 reps	8-10 reps	8-10 reps
Squat jump	6-8 reps	6-8 reps	8-10 reps	8-10 reps
Box crossover push-up	10-14 reps total	10-14 reps total	14-20 reps total	4-20 reps (total)
Stability-ball stir the pot	5-6 reps each side	5-6 reps each side	6-8 reps each side	6-8 reps (each side)
	Rest 2-3 min between sets.	Rest 2-3 min between sets.	Rest 1-2 rest between sets.	Rest 1-2 min between sets.
Unilateral farmer's walk complex	*2-3 rounds each side*	*2-3 rounds each side*	*2-3 rounds each side*	*2-3 rounds each side*
Farmer's walk (1 lap; right hand)	30-40 yd total	30-40 yd total	40-50 yd total	40-50 yd total
One-arm free-standing dumbbell row (left hand)	6-8 reps	6-8 reps	8-10 reps	8-10 reps
Farmer's walk (1 lap; right hand)	30-40 yd total	30-40 yd total	40-50 yd total	40-50 yd total
One-arm overhead push press (left hand)	6-8 reps	6-8 reps	8-10 reps	8-10 reps
Farmer's walk (1 lap; right hand)	30-40 yd total	30-40 yd total	40-50 yd total	40-50 yd total
Reverse lunge with dumbbell at shoulder (dumbbell in left hand; step back with left leg)	6-8 reps	6-8 reps	8-10 reps	8-10 reps
Farmer's walk (1 lap; right hand)	30-40 yds total	30-40 yds total	40-50 yds total	40-50 yd total
	Rest 30 sec before switching sides. Rest 2 min between rounds.	Rest 30 sec before switching sides. Rest 2 min between rounds.	Rest 30 sec before switching sides. Rest 2 min between rounds.	Rest 30 sec before switching sides. Rest 2 min between rounds.
Isolation exercises	*2-3 sets*	*2-3 sets*	*2-3 sets*	*2-3 sets*
Stability-ball leg curl	12-15 reps	12-15 reps	15-20 reps	15-20 reps
Ball back extension with arm Y	12-15 reps	12-15 reps	15-20 reps	15-20 reps
	Rest 60 sec between supersets.	Rest 60 sec between supersets.	Rest 60 sec between supersets.	Rest 60 sec between supersets.

Figure 9.5   Metabolic Strength Training Program 1: Workout B

	Week 1	Week 2	Week 3	Week 4
Angled barbell combination	*7 min (AMRAP)*	*8 min (AMRAP)*	*9 min (AMRAP)*	*9 min (AMRAP) (use a heavier load than week 3)*
Angled deadlift	1 rep	1 rep	1 rep	1 rep
Angled rotary press (switch sides every 3-6 reps)	1 rep	1 rep	1 rep	1 rep
	Rest 3-4 min.	Rest 3-4 min.	Rest 3-4 min.	Rest 3-4 min.
Big 4 circuit	*4-5 sets*	*4-5 sets*	*4-5 sets*	*4-5 sets*
Dumbbell uppercut	6-8 reps	6-8 reps	8-10 reps	8-10 reps
Dumbbell walking lunge	6-8 reps	6-8 reps	8-10 reps	8-10 reps
One-arm cable row	8-10 reps (each side)	8-10 reps (each side)	10-12 reps (each side)	10-12 reps (each side)
Ball knee tucks	10-14 reps (each side)	10-14 reps (each side)	14-20 reps (each side)	14-20 reps (each side)
	Rest 2-3 min between rounds.	Rest 2-3 min between rounds.	Rest 1-2 min between rounds.	Rest 1-2 min between rounds.
Dumbbell complex	*3-4 rounds (each side)*	*4-5 rounds (each side)*	*5-6 rounds (each side)*	*5-6 rounds (each side)*
Bent-over row	5-6 reps	6-7 reps	6-7 reps	7-8 reps
One-leg Romanian deadlift	5-6 reps (each side)	6-7 reps (each side)	6-7 reps (each side)	7-8 reps (each side)
Front squat	5-6 reps	6-7 reps	6-7 reps	7-8 reps
Push-up to plank row	6-8 reps	8-10 reps	8-10 reps	10-12 reps
	Rest 2-3 min between rounds.	Rest 2-3 min between rounds.	Rest 1-2 min between rounds.	Rest 1-2 min between rounds.
Isolation exercises	*2-3 sets*	*2-3 sets*	*2-3 sets*	*2-3 sets*
Cable high chop	8-10 reps (each side)	8-10 reps (each side)	10-12 reps (each side)	10-12 reps (each side)
Cable triceps rope extension	8-10 reps	8-10 reps	10-12 reps	10-12 reps
	Rest 60 sec between supersets.	Rest 60 sec between supersets.	Rest 60 sec between supersets.	Rest 60 sec between supersets.

Figure 9.6   Metabolic Strength Training Program 2: Workout A

	Week 1	Week 2	Week 3	Week 4
Kettlebell combination	8 min (AMRAP)	9 min (AMRAP)	10 min (AMRAP)	10 min (AMRAP) (use a heavier load than week 3)
Two-arm swing	2 reps	2 reps	2 reps	2 reps
Two-arm swing clean	1 rep	1 rep	1 rep	1 rep
Reverse lunge (each leg; kettlebells at shoulders)	1 rep (each leg)	1 rep (each leg)	1 rep (each leg)	1 rep (each leg)
Two-arm overhead push press	1 rep	1 rep	1 rep	1 rep
	Rest 3-4 min.	Rest 3-4 min.	Rest 2-3 min.	Rest 2-3 min.
Big 4 circuit	3-4 sets	3-4 sets	4-5 sets	4-5 sets
Dumbbell bench press	8-10 reps	8-10 reps	8-10 reps	8-10 reps
Lateral bound	6-8 reps (each side)	6-8 reps (each side)	6-8 reps (each side)	6-8 reps (each side)
One-arm dumbbell bench row	6-8 reps (each side)	6-8 reps (each side)	6-8 reps (each side)	6-8 reps (each side)
One-leg hip thrust	10-15 reps	10-15 reps	10-15 reps	10-15 reps
	Rest 2-3 min between rounds.	Rest 2-3 min between rounds.	Rest 1-2 min between rounds.	Rest 1-2 min between rounds.
Dumbbell complex	4 sets	4 sets	5 sets	5 sets
Uppercut	6-8 reps (each side)	6-8 reps (each side)	6-8 reps (each side)	6-8 reps (each side)
Front squat and Romanian deadlift	6-8 reps	6-8 reps	6-8 reps	6-8 reps
One-arm dumbbell bench row (each side)	6-8 reps (each side)	6-8 reps (each side)	6-8 reps (each side)	6-8 reps (each side)
	Rest 2-3 min between rounds.	Rest 2-3 min between rounds.	Rest 1-2 min between rounds.	Rest 1-2 min between rounds.
Isolation exercises	2-3 sets	2-3 sets	2-3 sets	2-3 sets
Hands-on-ball push-up (hands on box or med ball)	12-15 reps	12-15 reps	Max reps	Max reps
Stability-ball stir the pot	5-6 reps (each direction)	5-6 reps (each direction)	6-8 reps (each direction)	6-8 reps (each direction)
Ball back extension with arm Y	12-15 reps	12-15 reps	15-20 reps	15-20 reps
	Rest 60 sec between supersets.	Rest 60 sec between supersets.	Rest 60 sec between supersets.	Rest 60 sec between supersets.

Figure 9.7 Metabolic Strength Training Program 2: Workout B

	Week 1	Week 2	Week 3	Week 4
Dumbbell (unilateral) combination	8 min (AMRAP)	9 min (AMRAP)	10 min (AMRAP)	10 min (AMRAP) (use heavier load than week 3)
One-arm burpee	1 rep	1 rep	1 rep	1 rep
One-arm assisted hang clean	1 rep	1 rep	1 rep	1 rep
One-sided front squat with dumbbell at shoulder	1 rep	1 rep	1 rep	1 rep
One-arm uppercut (switch sides every 3-5 reps)	1 rep	1 rep	1 rep	1 rep
	Rest 3-4 min.	Rest 3-4 min.	Rest 3-4 min.	Rest 2-3 min.
Big 5 circuit	3-4 sets	3-4 sets	4-5 sets	4-5 sets
Machine lat pull-down (wide grip)	8-10 reps	8-10 reps	8-10 reps	8-10 reps
Dumbbell bench step-up	6-8 reps (each side)	6-8 reps (each side)	6-8 reps (each side)	6-8 reps (each side)
Push-back push-up	6-8 reps	6-8 reps	6-8 reps	6-8 reps
One-leg one-arm dumbbell Romanian deadlift	6-8 reps (each side)	6-8 reps (each side)	6-8 reps (each side)	6-8 reps (each side)
Ab snail	5-8 reps	5-8 reps	5-8 reps	5-8 reps
	Rest 2-3 min between rounds.	Rest 2-3 min between rounds.	Rest 1-2 min between rounds.	Rest 1-2 min between rounds.
Band complex	4 sets	4 sets	5 sets	5 sets
Lunge and band press	20-24 reps (total)	20-24 reps (total)	20-24 reps (total)	20-24 reps (total)
Band tight rotation	20-24 reps (each side)	20-24 reps (each side)	20-24 reps (each side)	20-24 reps (each side)
Split squat and one-arm row	10-12 reps (each side)	10-12 reps (each side)	10-12 reps (each side)	10-12 reps (each side)
	Rest 2-3 min between rounds.	Rest 2-3 min between rounds.	Rest 1-2 min between rounds.	Rest 1-2 min between rounds.
Isolation exercises	2-3 sets	2-3 sets	2-3 sets	2-3 sets
Suspension biceps curl	12-15 reps	12-15 reps	15-20 reps	15-20 reps
Wide-elbow suspension row	12-15 reps	12-15 reps	Max reps	Max reps
	Rest 60 sec between supersets.	Rest 60 sec between supersets.	Rest 60 sec between supersets.	Rest 60 sec between supersets.

Figure 9.8 Metabolic Strength Training Program 3: Workout A

	Week 1	Week 2	Week 3	Week 4
Dumbbell (unilateral) combination	*8 min (AMRAP)*	*9 min (AMRAP)*	*10 min (AMRAP)*	*10 min (AMRAP) (use heavier load than week 3)*
One-arm swing	2 reps	2 reps	2 reps	2 reps
One-arm assisted hang clean	1 rep	1 rep	1 rep	1 rep
One-sided front squat with dumbbell at shoulder	1 rep	1 rep	1 rep	1 rep
One-arm overhead push press (switch sides every 3-5 rounds through the complex)	1 rep	1 rep	1 rep	1 rep
	Rest 3-4 min.	Rest 3-4 min.	Rest 3-4 min.	Rest 2-3 min.
Big 4 circuit	*3-4 sets*	*3-4 sets*	*4-5 sets*	*4-5 sets*
Push-up lock-off	5-7 reps (each side)	5-7 reps (each side)	5-7 reps (each side)	5-7 reps (each side)
Barbell good morning	8-10 reps	8-10 reps	8-10 reps	8-10 reps
Barbell bent-over row (underhand grip)	6-8 reps	6-8 reps	6-8 reps	6-8 reps
Plank row	6-8 reps (each side)	6-8 reps (each side)	6-8 reps (each side)	6-8 reps (each side)
	Rest 2-3 min between rounds.	Rest 2-3 min between rounds.	Rest 1-2 min between rounds.	Rest 1-2 min between rounds.
Weight-plate complex	*3-4 sets*	*3-4 sets*	*4-5 sets*	*4-5 sets*
Diagonals	6-8 reps (each side)	6-8 reps (each side)	6-8 reps (each side)	6-8 reps (each side)
Middle chop	12-16 reps	12-16 reps	12-16 reps	12-16 reps
Lateral lunge	6-8 reps (each side)	6-8 reps (each side)	6-8 reps (each side)	6-8 reps (each side)
	Rest 2-3 min between rounds.	Rest 2-3 min between rounds.	Rest 1-2 min between rounds.	Rest 1-2 min between rounds.
Isolation exercises	*2-3 sets*	*2-3 sets*	*2-3 sets*	*2-3 sets*
Rear deltoid fly	12-15 reps	12-15 reps	15-20 reps	15-20 reps
Arm walk-out	4-6 reps	4-6 reps	6-8 reps	6-8 reps
	Rest 60 sec between supersets.	Rest 60 sec between supersets.	Rest 60 sec between supersets.	Rest 60 sec between supersets.

Figure 9.9   Metabolic Strength Training Program 3: Workout B

	Week 1	Week 2	Week 3	Week 4
Dumbbell (unilateral) combination				
Turkish get-up (alternate sides every 3 reps)	7 min (AMRAP); rest 3-4 min	8 min (AMRAP); rest 3-4 min	9 min (AMRAP); rest 3-4 min	9 min (AMRAP; use heavier load than week 3); rest 3-4 min
Big 4 circuit	*3-4 sets*	*3-4 sets*	*4-5 sets*	*4-5 sets*
Single-arm antirotation suspension row	8-10 reps (each side)	8-10 reps (each side)	8-10 reps (each side)	8-10 reps (each side)
Dumbbell Bulgarian split squat	6-8 reps (each side)	6-8 reps (each side)	6-8 reps (each side)	6-8 reps
Dumbbell bench press	6-8 reps	6-8 reps	6-8 reps	6-8 reps (each sided)
Band tight rotation	12-16 reps (each side)	12-16 reps (each side)	12-16 reps(each side)	12-16 reps (each side)
	Rest 2-3 min between rounds.	Rest 2-3 min between rounds.	Rest 1-2 min between rounds.	Rest 1-2 min between rounds.
Angled barbell complex	*3-4 sets*	*3-4 sets*	*4-5 sets*	*4-5 sets*
Reverse lunge	4-6 reps (each side)	4-6 reps (each side)	4-6 reps (each side)	4-6 reps (each side)
Angled shoulder-to-shoulder press	4-6 reps (each side)	4-6 reps (each side)	4-6 reps (each side)	4-6 reps (each side)
Angled deadlift to clean (left side)	6-8 reps	6-8 reps	6-8 reps	6-8 reps
Angled deadlift to clean (right side)	6-8 reps	6-8 reps	6-8 reps	6-8 reps
	Rest 2-3 min between rounds.	Rest 2-3 min between rounds.	Rest 1-2 min between rounds.	Rest 1-2 min between rounds.
Isolation exercises	*2-3 sets*	*2-3 sets*	*2-3 sets*	*2-3 sets*
Suspension triceps skull crusher	10-12 reps	10-12 reps	12-15 reps	12-15 reps
Suspension Y-pulls	10-12 reps	10-12 reps	12-15 reps	12-15 reps
	Rest 60 sec between supersets.	Rest 60 sec between supersets.	Rest 60 sec between supersets.	Rest 60 sec between supersets.

Figure 9.10   Metabolic Strength Training Program 4: Workout A

	Week 1	Week 2	Week 3	Week 4
Big circuit 3	*4-5 sets*	*4-5 sets*	*5-6 sets*	*5-6 sets*
Barbell Romanian deadlift	8-10 reps	8-10 reps	8-10 reps	8-10 reps
Pull-up	Max reps	Max reps	Max reps	Max reps
One-arm push-up	3-5 reps (each side)	3-5 reps (each side)	3-5 reps (each side)	3-5 reps (each side)
Big 4 (unilateral) circuit	*3-4 sets*	*3-4 sets*	*4-5 sets*	*4-5 sets*
Box crossover push-up	6-8 reps (each side)	6-8 reps (each side)	6-8 reps (each side)	6-8 reps (each side)
Knee-tap squat (body-weight or with dumbbells)	6-8 reps (each side)	6-8 reps (each side)	6-8 reps (each side)	6-8 res (each side)
One-arm free-standing dumbbell row	6-8 reps (each side)	6-8 reps (each side)	6-8 reps (each side)	6-8 reps (each side)
Dumbbell anterior-leaning lunge	6-8 reps (each side	6-8 reps (each side)	6-8 reps (each side)	6-8 reps (each side)
	Rest 2-3 min between rounds.	Rest 2-3 min between rounds.	Rest 1-2 min between rounds.	Rest 1-2 min between rounds.
Bilateral farmer's walk complex	*3-4 sets*	*3-4 sets*	*4-5 sets*	*4-5 sets*
Farmer's walk (1 lap)	30-40 yd	30-40 yd	30-40 yd	30-40 yd
Barbell bent-over rows	6-8 reps	6-8 reps	6-8 reps	6-8 reps
Farmer's walk (1 lap)	30-40 yd	30-40 yd	30-40 yd	30-40 yd
Dumbbell uppercut	4-6 reps (each side)	4-6 reps (each side)	4-6 reps (each side)	4-6 reps (each side)
Farmer's walk (1 lap)	30-40 yd	30-40 yd	30-40 yd	30-40 yd
Dumbbell reverse lunge (alternate legs)	5-6 reps (each side)	5-6 reps (each side)	5-6 reps (each side)	5-6 reps (each side)
Farmer's walk (1 lap)	30-40 yd	30-40 yd	30-40 yd	30-40 yd
	Rest 2-3 min between rounds.	Rest 2-3 min between rounds.	Rest 1-2 min between rounds.	Rest 1-2 min between rounds.
Isolation exercises	*2-3 sets*	*2-3 sets*	*2-3 sets*	*2-3 sets*
Cable biceps rope curl	12-15 reps	12-15 reps	15-20 reps	15-20 reps
Side plank to dumbbell lateral raise	8-10 reps (each side)	8-10 reps (each side)	10-12 reps (each side)	10-12 reps (each side)
	Rest 60 sec between supersets.	Rest 60 sec between supersets.	Rest 60 sec between supersets.	Rest 60 sec between supersets.

Figure 9.11 Metabolic Strength Training Program 4: Workout B

	Week 1	Week 2	Week 3	Week 4
Dumbbell combination	*8 min (AMRAP)*	*9 min (AMRAP)*	*10 min (AMRAP)*	*10 min (AMRAP)*
One-arm free-standing dumbbell row	1 rep	1 rep	1 rep	1 rep
Suitcase squat	2 reps	2 reps	2 reps	2 reps
One-arm assisted hang clean	1 rep	1 rep	1 rep	1 rep
One-arm overhead push press	1 rep (switch hands every 3-4 rounds)	1 rep (switch hands every 3-4 rounds)	1 rep (switch hands every 3-4 rounds)	1 rep (switch hands every 3-4 rounds)
	Rest 3-4 min.	Rest 3-4 min.	Rest 3-4 min.	Rest 3-4 min.
Band complex	*4 sets*	*4 sets*	*5 sets*	*5 sets*
Lunge and band press (alternate legs)	20-24 reps (total)	20-24 reps (total)	20-24 reps (total)	20-24 reps (total)
Band tight rotation	20-24 reps (each side)	20-24 reps (each side)	20-24 reps (each side)	20-24 reps (each side)
Band swimmers	20-24 reps	20-24 reps	20-24 reps	20-24 reps
One-arm compound row	10-12 reps (each side)	10-12 reps (each side)	10-12 reps (each side)	10-12 reps (each side)
	Rest 2-3 min between rounds.	Rest 2-3 min between rounds.	Rest 1-2 min between rounds.	Rest 1-2 min between rounds.
Body-weight countdown complex	*8 min (AMRAP)*	*9 min (AMRAP)*	*10 min (AMRAP)*	*10 min (AMRAP)*
Squat jump	4 reps	4 reps	4 reps	4 reps
Push-up	3 reps	3 reps	3 reps	3 reps
Burpee	2 reps	2 reps	2 reps	2 reps
Chin-up	1 rep	1 rep	1 rep	1 rep
	Rest 2-3 min between rounds.	Rest 2-3 min between rounds.	Rest 1-2 min between rounds.	Rest 1-2 min between rounds.
Isolation exercises	*2-3 sets*	*2-3 sets*	*2-3 sets*	*2-3 sets*
Ab snail	4-7 reps	4-7 reps	7-10 reps	7-10 reps
Barbell calf raise	12-15 reps	12-15 reps	15-20 reps	15-20 reps
	Rest 60 sec between supersets.	Rest 60 sec between supersets.	Rest 60 sec between supersets.	Rest 60 sec between supersets.

Figure 9.12 Metabolic Strength Training Program 5: Workout A

	Week 1	Week 2	Week 3	Week 4
Big 3 circuit	*4 sets*	*4 sets*	*5 sets*	*5 sets*
Pull-up	Max reps	Max reps	Max reps	Max reps
Dumbbell reverse lunge	6-8 reps (each side)	6-8 reps (each side)	6-8 reps (each side)	6-8 reps (each side)
Incline dumbbell press	6-8 reps	6-8 reps	6-8 reps	6-8 reps
	Rest 2-3 min between rounds.	Rest 2-3 min between rounds.	Rest 1-2 min between rounds.	Rest 1-2 min between rounds.
Big 5 circuit	*3-4 sets*	*3-4 sets*	*4-5 sets*	*4-5 sets*
Angled one-arm row	8-10 reps (each side)	8-10 reps (each side)	8-10 reps (each side)	8-10 reps (each side)
Knee-tap squat	6-8 reps (each side)	6-8 reps (each side)	6-8 reps (each side)	6-8 reps (each side)
Angled shoulder-to-shoulder press	6-8 reps (each side)	6-8 reps (each side)	6-8 reps (each side)	6-8 reps (each side)
One-arm swing	8-10 reps (each side)	8-10 reps (each side)	8-10 reps (each side)	8-10 reps (each side)
Arm walk-outs	3-5 reps	3-5 reps	3-5 reps	3-5 reps
	Rest 2-3 min between rounds.	Rest 2-3 min between rounds.	Rest 1-2 min between rounds.	Rest 1-2 min between rounds.
Weight-plate complex	*3-4 sets*	*3-4 sets*	*4-5 sets*	*4-5 sets*
Diagonal chop (each side)	8-10 reps (each side)	8-10 reps (each side)	8-10 reps (each side)	8-10 reps (each side)
Middle chop	10-12 reps	10-12 reps	10-12 reps	10-12 reps
Lateral lunge	6-8 reps (each side)	6-8 reps (each side)	6-8 reps (each side)	6-8 reps (each side)
Ball plate crunch	10-12 reps	10-12 reps	10-12 reps	10-12 reps
	Rest 2-3 min between rounds.	Rest 2-3 min between rounds.	Rest 1-2 min between rounds.	Rest 1-2 min between rounds.
Isolation exercises	*2-3 sets*	*2-3 sets*	*2-3 sets*	*2-3 sets*
One-leg hip thrust	12-15 reps (each side)	12-15 reps (each side)	15-20 reps (each side)	15-20 reps (each side)
Angled barbell tight rainbow	10-12 reps (each side)	10-12 reps (each side)	12-15 reps (each side)	12-15 reps (each side)
	Rest 60 sec between supersets.	Rest 60 sec between supersets.	Rest 60 sec between supersets.	Rest 60 sec between supersets.

Figure 9.13 Metabolic Strength Training Program 5: Workout B

	Week 1	Week 2	Week 3	Week 4
Big 4 circuit	*4 sets*	*4 sets*	*5 sets*	*5 sets*
Wide-grip bent-over row	8-10 reps	8-10 reps	8-10 reps	8-10 reps
Dumbbell anterior-leaning lunge	6-8 reps (each side)	6-8 reps (each side)	6-8 reps (each side)	6-8 reps (each side)
Dumbbell bench press	8-10 reps	8-10 reps	8-10 reps	8-10 reps
One-arm dumbbell uppercut	6-8 reps (each side)	6-8 reps (each side)	6-8 reps (each side)	6-8 reps (each side)
	Rest 2-3 min between rounds.	Rest 2-3 min between rounds.	Rest 1-2 min between rounds.	Rest 1-2 min between rounds.
Big 4 circuit	*3-4 sets*	*3-4 sets*	*4-5 sets*	*4-5 sets*
Bulgarian split squat	6-8 reps (each side)	6-8 reps (each side)	6-8 reps (each side)	6-8 reps (each side)
Dumbbell plank row	6-8 reps (each side)	6-8 reps (each side)	6-8 reps (each side)	6-8 reps (each side)
Squat to Romanian deadlift	6-8 reps	6-8 reps	6-8 reps	6-8 reps
Dumbbell bench press	6-8 reps	6-8 reps	6-8 reps	6-8 reps
	Rest 2-3 min between rounds.	Rest 2-3 min between rounds.	Rest 1-2 min between rounds.	Rest 1-2 min between rounds.
Two kettlebell combination (one in each hand)	*8 min (AMRAP)*	*9 min (AMRAP)*	*10 min (AMRAP)*	*10 min (AMRAP) (use a heavier load than week 3)*
Two-arm swing	2 reps	2 reps	2 reps	2 reps
Two-arm swing clean	1 rep	1 rep	1 rep	1 rep
Front squat	1 rep	1 rep	1 rep	1 rep
Two-arm overhead push press	1 rep	1 rep	1 rep	1 rep
Isolation exercises	*2-3 sets*	*2-3 sets*	*2-3 sets*	*2-3 sets*
Cable high chop	8-10 reps (each side)	8-10 reps (each side)	12-15 reps (each side)	12-15 reps (each side)
Ball back extension with arm Y	12-15 reps	12-15 reps	12-15 reps	12-15 reps
	Rest 60 sec between supersets.	Rest 60 sec between supersets.	Rest 60 sec between supersets.	Rest 60 sec between supersets.

Figure 9.14   Metabolic Strength Training Program 6: Workout A

	Week 1	Week 2	Week 3	Week 4
Big 4 circuit	*4 sets*	*4 sets*	*5 sets*	*5 sets*
Dumbbell bench press	10-12 reps	10-12 reps	10-12 reps	10-12 reps
One-leg one-arm dumbbell Romanian deadlift (alternate legs)	6-8 reps (each side)	6-8 reps (each side)	6-8 reps (each side)	6-8 reps (each side)
Wide-grip seated row	10-12 reps	10-12 reps	10-12 reps	10-12 reps
Ball pike rollback	8-10 reps	8-10 reps	8-10 reps	8-10 reps
	Rest 2-3 min between rounds.	Rest 2-3 min between rounds.	Rest 1-2 min between rounds.	Rest 1-2 min between rounds.
Big 4 circuit	*3-4 sets*	*3-4 sets*	*4-5 sets*	*4-5 sets*
Dumbbell bench step-up	6-8 reps (each side)	6-8 reps (each side)	6-8 reps (each side)	6-8 reps (each side)
T-bar row	8-10 reps	8-10 reps	8-10 reps	8-10 reps
Dumbbell anterior lunges	6-8 reps (each side)	6-8 reps (each side)	6-8 reps (each side)	6-8 reps (each side)
Box crossover push-up	6-8 reps (each side)	6-8 reps (each side)	6-8 reps (each side)	6-8 reps (each side)
	Rest 2-3 min between rounds.	Rest 2-3 min between rounds.	Rest 1-2 min between rounds.	Rest 1-2 min between rounds.
Big 4 circuit	*3-4 sets*	*3-4 sets*	*4-5 sets*	*4-5 sets*
One-arm compound row	8-10 reps (each side)	8-10 reps (each side)	8-10 reps (each side)	8-10 reps (each side)
Squat jump	8-10 reps	8-10 reps	8-10 reps	8-10 reps
One-arm cable press	8-10 reps	8-10 reps	8-10 reps	8-10 reps
Stability-ball leg curl	15-20 reps	15-20 reps	15-20 reps	15-20 reps
	Rest 2-3 min between rounds.	Rest 2-3 min between rounds.	Rest 1-2 min between rounds.	Rest 1-2 min between rounds.
Isolation exercises	*2-3 sets*	*2-3 sets*	*2-3 sets*	*2-3 sets*
Angled barbell tight rainbow	12-15 reps (each side)	12-15 reps (each side)	15-20 reps (each side)	15-20 reps (each side)
Triceps dumbbell skull crusher	12-15 reps	12-15 reps	15-20 reps	15-20 reps
	Rest 60 sec between supersets.	Rest 60 sec between supersets.	Rest 60 sec between supersets.	Rest 60 sec between supersets.

Figure 9.15 Metabolic Strength Training Program 6: Workout B

	Week 1	Week 2	Week 3	Week 4
Barbell combination	8 min (as fast as possible)	9 min (as fast as possible)	10 min (as fast as possible)	10 min (AMRAP) (use a heavier load than week 3)
Bent-over row	1 rep	1 rep	1 rep	1 rep
Romanian deadlift	2 rep	2 rep	2 rep	2 rep
Jump shrug	1 rep	1 rep	1 rep	1 rep
Clean	1 rep	1 rep	1 rep	1 rep
Overhead push press	1 rep	1 rep	1 rep	1 rep
Front squat	1 rep	1 rep	1 rep	1 rep
	Rest 3-4 min.	Rest 3-4 min.	Rest 2-3 min.	Rest 2-3 min.
Body-weight countdown complex	8 min (AMRAP)	9 min (AMRAP)	10 min (AMRAP)	10 min (AMRAP) (use a heavier load than week 3)
Overhead reverse lunge	4 reps (each leg)	4 reps (each leg)	4 reps (each leg)	4 reps (each leg)
Break-dancer push-up	3 reps	3 reps	3 reps	3 reps
Frog jump	2 reps	2 reps	2 reps	2 reps
Chin-up	1 rep	1 rep	1 rep	1 rep
	Rest 2-3 min between rounds.	Rest 2-3 min between rounds.	Rest 1-2 min between rounds.	Rest 1-2 min between rounds.
Unilateral farmer's walk complex	3-4 sets (each side)	3-4 sets (each side)	4-5 sets (each side)	4-5 sets (each side)
Farmer's walk (1 lap; right hand)	30-40 yds	30-40 yds	30-40 yds	30-40 yds
One-arm swing (left hand)	6-8 reps	6-8 reps	6-8 reps	6-8 reps
Farmer's walk 1 lap; right hand)	30-40 yds	30-40 yds	30-40 yds	30-40 yds
Reverse lunge (dumbbell in left hand; step back with left leg)	6-8 reps	6-8 reps	6-8 reps	6-8 reps
Farmer's walk (1 lap; right hand)	30-40 yds	30-40 yds	30-40 yds	30-40 yds
One-leg Romanian deadlift (dumbbell in left hand; stand on right leg)	6-8 reps	6-8 reps	6-8 reps	6-8 reps
Farmer's walk (1 lap; right hand)	30-40 yds	30-40 yds	30-40 yds	30-40 yds
	Rest 2-3 min between rounds.	Rest 2-3 min between rounds.	Rest 1-2 min between rounds.	Rest 1-2 min between rounds.
Isolation exercises	2-3 sets	2-3 sets	2-3 sets	2-3 sets
Band tight rotation	12-15 reps (each side)	12-15 reps (each side)	15-20 reps (each side)	15-20 reps (each side)
Cable triceps rope extension	12-15 reps	12-15 reps	15-20 reps	15-20 reps
	Rest 60 sec between supersets.	Rest 60 sec between supersets.	Rest 60 sec between supersets.	Rest 60 sec between supersets.

Setting Up Your Weekly Metabolic Strength Training Program

To help you set up your weekly metabolic strength training program, let's assume you train 4 days per week. Here are a few options.

Figure 9.16
Four-Day Weekly Training: Option 1

Monday	Workout A
Tuesday	Workout B
Wednesday	Rest or active rest (see chapter 10)
Thursday	Workout A
Friday	Workout B
Saturday	Rest or active rest
Sunday	Rest or active rest

Figure 9.17
Four-Day Weekly Training: Option 2

Monday	Rest or active rest (see chapter 10)
Tuesday	Workout A
Wednesday	Workout B
Thursday	Rest or active rest
Friday	Workout A
Saturday	Workout B
Sunday	Rest or active rest

Figure 9.18
Four-Day Weekly Training: Option 3

Monday	Workout A
Tuesday	Rest or active rest (see chapter 10)
Wednesday	Workout B
Thursday	Rest or active rest
Friday	Workout A
Saturday	Workout B
Sunday	Rest or active rest

BODY-WEIGHT WORKOUT PROGRAMS

If you can't always make it to the gym, you can use the following workout programs that use only body-weight and band exercises (see figures 9.19a and 9.19b). These workouts are intended to be used only as an addition to your regular weekly gym-based workouts, on days when you're traveling, can't make it into the gym, or when you don't have access to a gym.

In other words, these body-weight workout programs are *not* intended to be done exclusively and they are *not* designed to replace you gym-based workouts; your primary training should be done using equipment. However, it's fine to occasionally substitute one or a few of these body-weight programs even when you can get to the gym simply to mix things up with your training.

There are two body-weight workouts provided: Workout A is intermediate level and workout B is advanced. Choose the workout that best fits your fitness level. Feel free to alternate the two workouts, or stick with the same workout two or three times before switching to the other one and performing it two or three times.

Both body-weight workouts are designed to be performed as circuits. Perform exercises labeled as *1a*, *1b*, and *1c* back to back, and rest after you've completed all the exercises within a given circuit. If needed, rest as little as you need, as much as you have to between exercises. Repeat the same exercises (i.e., the same circuit) for the number of sets indicated. Then repeat with exercises labeled as *2a*, *2b*, *2c*, and so on. Rest 60-90 seconds between circuits.

Figure 9.19*a* Body-Weight Workout Program A

MINI-CIRCUIT 1 (2-3 SETS)	
1a. Squat jump	8-10 reps
1b. Break-dancer push-up	8-10 reps
1c. Band lat pull-down	12-15 reps
MINI-CIRCUIT 2 (2-3 SETS)	
2a. Bulgarian split squat	10-12 reps (each side)
2b. Push-back push-up	10-15 reps
2c. Band swimmers	15-20 reps
MINI-CIRCUIT 3 (2-3 SETS)	
3a. One-leg hip thrust	12-15 reps (each side)
3b. Lunge and band press	16-20 reps (total)
3c. Split squat and row	12-15 reps (each side)
PAIRED SETS (2-3 SETS)	
4a. Band high-chop	12-15 reps (each side)
4b. Arm walk-out	4-6 reps
BODY-WEIGHT COMPLEX (1-2 SETS COMPLETED AS FAST AS POSSIBLE)	
5a. One-arm compound row	15 reps (each side)
5b. Overhead reverse lunge	16 reps (total)
5c. Push-up	8-10 reps
5d. Burpee	10-15 reps

Figure 9.19*b* Body-Weight Workout Program B

MINI-CIRCUIT 1 (2-3 SETS)	
1a. Anterior-leaning lunge scissor jump	8-10 reps (total)
1b. Break-dancer push-up	8-10 reps
1c. One-leg hip thrust	10-15 (each side)
1d. One-arm compound band row	12-15 reps (each side)
MINI-CIRCUIT 2 (2-3 SETS)	
2a. Knee-tap squat	10-12 reps (each side)
2b. Push-back push-up	10-15 reps
2c. Band swimmers	15-20 reps
2d. Chop	10-15 reps (each side)
MINI-CIRCUIT 3 (2-3 SETS)	
3a. Lateral bound	12-15 reps (each side)
3b. Lunge and band press	16-20 reps (total)
3c. Alternate-arm band row	24-30 reps (each stance)
3d. Ab snail	4-6 reps
BODY-WEIGHT COMPLEX (2-4 SETS COMPLETED AS FAST AS POSSIBLE)	
4a. Arm walk-out	5 reps
4b. Split-squat scissor jump	16 reps (total)
4c. Break-dancer push-up	8-10 reps
4d. Burpee—frog jump	8-10 reps

FAT-LOSS FIVE WORKOUT PROGRAM

The Fat-Loss Five workout is a plug-and-play training formula that builds on the circuit training concepts covered in chapter 4. Plus, the name *Fat-Loss Five* is cool, catchy, and easy to remember.

Put simply, a Fat-Loss Five sequence consists of five exercises performed back to back in a circuit. This circuit is developed to not only be a simple (but not easy) training formula to follow, it's also designed to be a fully comprehensive training formula that covers all of the bases. There are two basic components to the Fat-Loss Five circuit: four strength exercises and one total-body cardio exercise.

While you're cycling through strength exercises, the sequencing of the Fat-Loss Five circuit creates a constant cardiorespiratory effect. Whenever you perform any strength exercise, your body pumps more blood to the muscles involved in the movement. By performing an upper-body exercise, followed by a lower-body exercise, followed by a core exercise, you're constantly changing where your body must increase blood flow. Additionally, finishing each circuit of strength exercises with a burst of total-body cardio interval exercise keeps this cardiorespiratory effect going even longer.

Here are the five categories that make up a Fat-Loss Five circuit:

1. Upper-body pushing exercise
2. Upper-body pulling exercise
3. Lower-body leg- or hip-oriented exercise
4. Core exercise
5. Cardio exercise

The beauty of the Fat-Loss Five circuit is its simplicity and versatility. You can plug in virtually any exercise you want as long as it fits in the five categories. For the strength training exercises, any of the movements (using free weights or body weight) from the circuits chapter can be used in a Fat-Loss Five circuit. Additionally, any of the body-weight exercises from the chapter on body-weight

training can also be integrated into Fat-Loss Five circuits as long as they fit into one of the five strength-based movement categories just listed. Following is more detail on each of the categories.

Upper-Body Pushing Exercise

The purpose of these exercises is to incorporate the muscles of the chest, shoulders, triceps, and torso in order to maintain a stable body position. Here's a list of the top five exercises I suggest for this category:

1. Lunge and band press
2. Break-dancer push-up
3. Push-back push-up
4. Box crossover push-up
5. Uppercut (with dumbbells)

Upper-Body Pulling Exercise

The purpose of these exercises is to incorporate the muscles of the back, shoulders, biceps, and torso in order to maintain a stable body position. Here's a list of the top five exercises I suggest for this category:

1. Wide-grip band row
2. Band swimmers
3. Alternate-arm band rows
4. Suspension rows (low elbow or wide elbow)
5. Suspension Y-pulls

Lower-Body Exercise

You can choose either a leg-oriented or hip-oriented lower-body exercise to fill this category. The purpose of these exercises is to incorporate the muscles of the legs, glutes, and torso in order to maintain a stable body position. Here's a list of the top five exercises I suggest for this category:

1. Front or back squat (with barbell)
2. Swing (with kettlebell or dumbbell)
3. Lateral lunge
4. Frog jump
5. Alternate-leg step-up (with dumbbell)

Core Exercise

The purpose of these exercises is to focus on the abdominal and oblique musculature while also incorporating the hips and shoulders, which, as mentioned earlier, has been shown to be a more effective way of training the abdominal muscles compared with trying to isolate them. Here's a list of the top five exercises I suggest for this category:

1. Ab snail
2. Arm walk-out
3. Stability-ball knee tuck
4. Angled barbell rainbow
5. One-arm plank

Cardio Exercise

Several options for cardio exercises in the Fat-Loss Five circuit are provided here. Although we don't recommend using these exercises as long-duration, steady-state cardio in the workout programs provided in this book, they are added in short duration within Fat-Loss Five circuits to boost their effectiveness. They are kept to short 1- to 2-minute intervals, which drastically reduces the impact on your joints that they create when performed for extended lengths of time. The cardio options for the Fat-Loss Five include shadowboxing or kickboxing, rope jumping, running, stationary bike (Airdyne bike is preferred), rower, reaction ball, elliptical trainer, and VersaClimber.

Fat-Loss Five Protocol

A full Fat-Loss Five circuit is 4 minutes of total work time with 1 minute of rest time (5 minutes total). Thus, 2 rounds last a total of 10 minutes and 3 rounds last a total of 15 minutes. Now you can see where the name Fat-Loss Five comes from: There are five exercises and each circuit takes exactly 5 minutes. Also, as you'll see in the workouts later in this chapter, you'll typically perform 2 to 3 rounds of a given Fat-Loss Five circuit.

Each of the four strength exercises in a Fat-Loss Five circuit is performed for 30 seconds. You then rest 15 seconds before starting the next strength-based exercise. However, the total-body cardio interval, which is done last, is performed for 1 to 2 minutes. This means that as you become fitter, you may not need to take a complete rest for 60 seconds between circuits. Instead, you may want to do a longer active recovery by extending your cardio interval to 2 minutes (instead of 1 minute) and then going directly into your next circuit. In other words, you never stop moving. It's still 5 minutes either way you spin it; you do a minute of cardio and take a minute break before you start your next circuit round, or you do 2 minutes of cardio and then start your next circuit round. Of course, eliminating full rest breaks will make your workouts even more productive because you're doing more activity in the same time frame.

Fat-Loss Five and Bilateral Exercises

Although unilateral exercises can certainly be implemented within a Fat-Loss Five circuit as described in the circuits chapter, these circuits run smoother when they use purely bilateral exercises or alternating-limb exercises such as lunges or step-ups (where you switch legs on each rep). Also, compound movements (e.g., squats, push-ups, chin-ups, barbell rows) are better in Fat-Loss Five circuits instead of smaller, single-joint exercises (e.g., biceps curls, triceps extensions). Compound movements create a better metabolic training response than single-joint actions because they involve more muscles, and the goal of the Fat-Loss Five protocol is to maximize the metabolic effect of every rep, every circuit sequence, and every workout.

There are two intensities to consider for the Fat-Loss Five circuit: the total intensity of the entire circuit and the working intensity of each exercise within a given circuit. During the strength exercises within a circuit, you should be able to complete the entire 30 seconds of work time with good exercise form and at a fairly consistent tempo from what you started with. On a scale of 1 to 10 (with 10 being working very hard), at the end of each strength exercise you should be working at around a 7 or 8. Also, because the strength exercises are performed at a higher intensity than the total-body cardio exercise, they're performed for a shorter amount of time (30 seconds). The goal is to complete as many reps as you can within the 30 seconds. However, never sacrifice movement quality for quantity. If fatigue begins to interfere with your quality of movement (i.e., exercise form), simply perform your reps more slowly or reduce the range of motion (e.g., don't go as deep on squats or push-ups) in order to make the exercises easier and more manageable to maintain proper control.

For the cardio interval, use a pace that gets you at or around 70 to 80 percent of your max heart rate. By the time you're about to begin the next round of the circuit, you should feel mostly recovered. If you can get out a full sentence without breathing heavily (huffing and puffing), you're good to go into your next round. But, if you're still sucking wind after a 60-second break between circuits, you need to reduce the intensity of your cardio interval.

After you've performed 2 to 3 rounds of the same exercises in a given Fat-Loss Five circuit, the strength exercises change but the cardio exercise remains consistent throughout the entire workout, no matter how many times the strength exercises change. Keeping the cardio drill the same allows you to develop a consistent rhythm throughout the workout, while changing the strength moves every 2 to 3 rounds creates enough variety to keep things interesting and helps stimulate your muscles in a variety of ways.

Fat-Loss Five Workouts

Figure 9.20 offers two Fat-Loss Five workouts—one intermediate and one advanced. Be sure to choose the correct workout for your fitness level. Feel free to mix up the exercises you use in the strength or cardio portion of your circuits. Just make sure to stick with the circuit structure.

Figure 9.20a   Fat-Loss Five Workout Program A

FAT-LOSS FIVE CIRCUIT 1 (2-3 SETS*)	
1a. Prisoner squat	30 sec
1b. One-arm plank	15 sec (each side)
1c. Push-up with T-roll	30 sec
1d. Alternate-arm band row	30 sec (15 sec each stance)
Cardio: shadowboxing	1 min
FAT-LOSS FIVE CIRCUIT 2 (2-3 SETS*)	
2a. Anterior lunge (with dumbbells)	30 sec (total)
2b. Arm walk-out	30 sec
2c. Lunge and band press	30 sec
2d. Wide-grip band row	30 sec
Cardio: shadowboxing	1 min
FAT-LOSS FIVE CIRCUIT 3 (2-3 SETS*)	
3a. Lateral lunge	30 sec (total)
3b. Standing anti-rotation band press	15 sec (each side)
3c. Ball push-up	30 sec
3d. Band swimmer	30 sec
Cardio: shadowboxing	1 min

*Rest 15 sec. between exercises and 1 min. between sets.

Figure 9.20*b* Fat-Loss Five Workout Program B

FAT-LOSS FIVE CIRCUIT 1 (2-3 SETS*)	
1a. 2 squats (body weight) alternated with 1 burpee	30 sec
1b. Break-dancer push-up	30 sec
1c. Alternate-arm band row	30 sec (15 sec each stance)
1d. Band tight rotation	30 sec (15 sec each stance)
Cardio: rope jumping	1 min
FAT-LOSS FIVE CIRCUIT 2 (2-3 SETS*)	
2a. Anterior lunge (with dumbbells)	30 sec
2b. Arm walk-out	30 sec
2c. Lunge and band press	30 sec
Cardio: shadowboxing	1 min
FAT-LOSS FIVE CIRCUIT 3 (2-3 SETS*)	
3a. Rotational lunge	30 sec total
3b. Ab snail	30 sec
3c. Push-back push-up with twist	30 sec
3d. Band lat pull-down	30 sec
Cardio: rope jumping	1 min
FAT-LOSS FIVE CIRCUIT 4 (2-3 SETS*)	
4a. Step-up (with dumbbells)	30 sec total
4b. Plank row (with dumbbells)	15 sec (each side)
4c. Two-arm compound band row	30 sec
4d. Dumbbell uppercut	30 sec
Cardio: shadowboxing	1 min

*Rest 15 sec. between exercises and 1 min. between sets.

Adding a Fat-Loss Five Workout to Weekly Training

The workout method described in the previous section also gives you the option of using the Fat-Loss Five protocol on one of your training days to add more variety to your programs and make your workouts more diverse. If your schedule allows you to train 5 days a week, following are several 5-day weekly training plans that incorporate one Fat-Loss Five training day.

If your schedule allows you to train 5 days a week, which is preferred for best results, following are some 5-day weekly training plans that incorporate one Fat-Loss Five training day.

Figure 9.21 Four-Day Weekly Training With Fat-Loss Five: Option 1*

Monday	Workout A
Tuesday	Workout B
Wednesday	Rest or active rest
Thursday	Workout A
Friday	Fat-Loss Five workout (45 min)
Saturday	Rest or active rest
Sunday	Rest or active rest

*Begin the following week using workout B on Monday, workout A on Tuesday, and so on.

Figure 9.22
Four-Day Weekly Training With Fat-Loss Five: Option 2*

Monday	Rest or active rest
Tuesday	Workout A
Wednesday	Workout B
Thursday	Rest or active rest
Friday	Workout A
Saturday	Fat-Loss Five workout (45 min)
Sunday	Rest or active rest

*Begin the following week using workout B on Tuesday, workout A on Wednesday, and so on.

Figure 9.23
Four-Day Weekly Training With Fat-Loss Five: Option 3*

Monday	Workout A
Tuesday	Rest or active rest
Wednesday	Workout B
Thursday	Rest or active rest
Friday	Workout A
Saturday	Fat-Loss Five workout (45 min)
Sunday	Rest or active rest

*Begin the following week using workout B on Monday, workout A on Wednesday, and so on.

Figure 9.24
Five-Day Weekly Training With Fat-Loss Five: Option 1

Monday	Workout A
Tuesday	Workout B
Wednesday	Rest or active rest
Thursday	Workout A
Friday	Workout B
Saturday	Fat-Loss Five workout (35-50 min)
Sunday	Rest or active rest

Figure 9.25
Five-Day Weekly Training With Fat-Loss Five: Option 2

Monday	Rest or active rest
Tuesday	Workout A
Wednesday	Workout B
Thursday	Rest or active rest
Friday	Workout A
Saturday	Workout B
Sunday	Fat-Loss Five workout (35-50 min)

Now that you've been given the meat and potatoes, it's time for dessert. In the next chapter we will cover some things you should know in order to continue to benefit from the training strategies provided in this book for a long time to come.

chapter 100

Fat-Loss Training for Life

The goal of this final chapter is to provide a variety of simple and practical lifestyle strategies. These strategies will help you not just get results in the short term from the workout concepts and programs in this book but also maintain long-term, sustainable results.

CHANGE UP YOUR ROUTINE

One of the beauties of the human body is that it's adaptive. The more it does something, the better and more efficient it becomes at doing it. Although this is a wonderful quality that allows us to improve the things we practice, it also means that the more we do a specific workout, the less likely that a particular workout is to be as beneficial as it was when we first started doing it. However, there also has to be some consistency in the workouts you do so that you can ensure that you practice specific (new) exercises to improve your skill at performing them and create neural adaptions, which allow you to better coordinate the activation of all relevant muscles working in a given exercise.[1] Not to mention, also improving your fitness level based on the demands of the program. In other words, if you are constantly changing your workouts, you have no way of gauging if you are getting better.

So yes, you want variety in your training, but not too much, too often. Let's explore how your body adapts to exercise and how often I recommend changing your routine.

Understand How Your Body Reacts to Exercise

One of the most common questions about training is how often you should change your workouts. The answer I give to this is every 3 to 5 weeks, which is based on Hans Selye's general adaptation syndrome (GAS). GAS describes three stages of the human body's response to stress.

Alarm, or Shock

This stage involves the initial shock of the new stimulus to the system, which can include muscle soreness, stiffness, and possible (temporary) drops in performance. This first stage is unavoidable; it will happen every time (early on) you switch your program every 3 to 5 weeks.

Resistance, or Adaptation

This stage involves a positive adaptation by the body to the stimulus, which can include increased muscle size and strength, improved motor unit recruitment (i.e., neuromuscular coordination), and increased connective tissue strength and bone mass. The goal is to create a positive *adaptation* to the new program (i.e., training stimulus) without reaching the point of *accommodation*, where you stop positively adapting.

Changing your program every 3 to 5 weeks gives your body enough time to adapt; improved neuromuscular coordination and increased muscle hypertrophy (i.e., muscle size) have been shown to occur in early stages (the first 3-5 weeks) or when starting new training program (2,3,4), but isn't long enough for your body to accommodate to the training stimulus where the program becomes stale and is much less or no longer beneficial. If you're doing the same reps each week, it's a good idea to change the exercises you use more often, around every 3 to 4 weeks. However, if you're changing the amount of sets and reps you use each week for the same exercises, you don't have to change your program as often due to the variety in repetitions. So, changing your program every 5 to 6 weeks is in order.

Exhaustion, or Fatigue

This stage involves a decrease in the body's ability to repair and to positively respond to stress, which can lead to overtraining, boredom, and reductions in performance and energy. You want to avoid the exhaustion stage where you're doing more in your training than your body can handle.

Use the Same Exercises in Different Ways

Speaking of your body adapting to exercise, any good program should have enough consistency to allow you to see progress, and it should have enough variety to prevent boredom and potential repetitive stress injury. This involves using the same basic exercises but in slightly different ways. For example, with a squat, you can mix up your foot positions (wider stance or parallel stance), you can place the bar in various positions (e.g., front squat, back squat, trap bar), and you can perform single-leg versions such as split squats and knee-tap squats. The consistent exercise is the squat, but every few weeks you perform a different squat variation like the ones just described. There's no need to try to get too crazy and fancy with exercises. As with anything in life, it's focusing on the basics (e.g., squat) and knowing how to make the most out of the basic movements (e.g., squat variations) that's going to make your training successful.

Personalize Your Exercises

One of the biggest mistakes in working out—and personal trainers often make this mistake—is attempting to fit the individual to the exercises instead of fitting the exercises to the individual. All of us are the same species, human, just like all automobiles are the same type of vehicle. But just like automobiles, humans come in all shapes and sizes. Just as you would never expect a brand-new sports car to drive and handle the same as a brand-new work truck, it's unrealistic to expect a guy who's built like a football running back to move the same as a guy who is built like a football lineman. It only makes sense that although both the running back and lineman can squat, push, twist, pull, and so on, they may perform the movements in slightly different ways. In other words, there is not any exact exercise that matches the movement of everyone, because there are variations in the way individual humans move. Therefore, people must choose the particular exercise variations that best fit how they move.

Not only do we all move a bit differently based on our size and shape, which is dictated by our own unique skeletal framework and body proportions, but past injury, loss of cartilage, or natural joint degenerative processes such as arthritis can influence how we move. So, attempting to fit every person to the same exercise movement is potentially dangerous. Doing so could cause a problem or further exacerbate an existing problem because it may go against one's current physiology and movement capability.

Trying to fit yourself to certain exercises simply doesn't make any sense from either a physiological or safety standpoint. That said, here's a simple way to find exercises that do make sense, because it takes an individualized approach to exercise selection.

This book has provided five categories of exercises that should be included in all training programs to ensure your workouts are fully comprehensive: upper-body pushing, upper-body pulling, lower-body leg oriented, lower-body hip oriented, and abdominal or core. Within each of these categories, you've been given a large variety of exercise options to choose from. When it comes to choosing the exercises that best fit you, there are two simple criteria:

1. *Comfort*—The movement is pain free, feels natural, works within your current physiology, and so on.

2. *Control*—You can demonstrate the movement technique and body positioning as provided in each exercise description. For example, when squatting, you display good knee and spinal alignment throughout, along with smooth, deliberate movement.

To allow for comfort and control, you may have to modify (shorten) the range of motion of a particular exercise, such as a squat to best fit your current ability. As discussed earlier, you should perform the workouts for roughly 4 weeks to make sure you can gauge your progress based on the last time you did the workout. The way to gauge your progress can be summarized in one word: performance!

Improvements in your performance can show up as increases in exercise range of motion (e.g., your squat depth improves) or as improvements in strength. Improvements in strength are obvious in that you lift more weight or perform more reps using the same weight load than you did previously.

In regard to gauging your exercise range of motion, if you did lose some movement range of motion from simply not using it (i.e., if you don't use it, you lose it), that lost range of motion gradually comes back once you reinstate the movement (i.e., exercise) into your regular lifestyle. And, if your range of motion does not improve, or if it ceases to improve in a given movement once you've been regularly performing that movement (with good comfort and control, of course),

it's not recommended that you push yourself to go further because you're probably already using what your physiology currently allows.

Learn How to Train Hard and Smart

Many of the metabolic strength training concepts in this book are high intensity and therefore challenging. As excited as you may be to get after it and put these workouts into practice, understand that, as you learned earlier, in order for a workout program to be maximally safe and effective, you must avoid the exhaustion (i.e., fatigue) stage. The "go hard or go home" mentality isn't the smartest approach to training; instead, it's an ego-driven recipe for quickly reducing your performance and health.

Be sure to begin using the concepts in this book by using your brain, not your ego. Progress through the workouts at a gradual pace, keeping all of your workouts at a level that challenges your current fitness without leaving you crawling on the floor or feeling like you want you throw up. Any type of training can make you tired, but only smart training can make you better. Be smart and don't judge your workouts by the fatigue they create, judge them by the results they create, which is more muscle and less body fat (without injury).

Incorporate Other Types of Exercise

You've been given a large variety of exercise options to include in your metabolic strength training workouts. We've also discussed the importance of using a variety of exercises to not only fit how your body moves but also to keep your workouts interesting and to keep your body positively adapting. That being said, although all of the exercises in this book are different, they can still be grouped under the same type of training, which is (metabolic) strength training. And, just as it's important to do a variety of exercises to ensure your workouts are comprehensive, it's also important to incorporate diversity in the type of exercise you do to ensure you develop a body that's not only lean but also well rounded in its abilities. Following are various types of exercise that can diversify and complement your metabolic strength training.

Take Up a Sport

What's the difference between running sprints and running football pass patterns with someone playing quarterback and throwing to you? Actually, they're virtually the same, but sprinting to catch a football is way more fun because it's playing, whereas running sprints is "working out." Regardless of how motivated you are to exercise, physical activity is more fun when it's done as part of a game. Taking up a sport that you regularly play and practicing a few times per week will not only help you stay more active, which will help keep you lean and fit, but it can also be more fun than just going to gym. Plus, it will serve as a tremendous complement to the metabolic strength training programs in this book.

Take Up Yoga

The general rule of joints is that they're designed to primarily function in their midranges of motion, but they also need some full range-of-motion activity in order to stay healthy and maintain their current range of motion. And, again, "If you don't use it, you lose it," as the saying goes.

The metabolic strength training concepts in this book avoid end-range joint actions, which is the safest way to lift heavy loads. That said, attending a yoga class one or more times per week can serve as a nice complement to your metabolic strength training workouts. Because of its low-load, slow-paced nature, many yoga moves require your joints to move into their end-range of motion, moving them in a manner that you don't get from weight training. Doing yoga can help to ensure better joint health, provide more variety of activity, and give you a more well-rounded body that's not just strong and lean but also mobile. In addition, many athletes have found yoga to be helpful for improving their ability to relax and recover from intense exercise.

TAKE TIME FOR REST AND RECOVERY

Taking time to rest and recover from intense exercise such as the metabolic strength workouts in this book is vital because your body does not grow stronger and fitter while you're working out; it improves and grows stronger in the recovery period between your workouts. So, improving your recovery will improve your results. This is one of the main reasons why the workout programs in this book recommend performing metabolic strength training four to five times per week. This ensures you get ample time to recover between workouts, minimize risk of overtraining, and continue to make gains.

Recognize Pain

This should be obvious, but many people are stubborn and use exercises that cause them pain. As stated earlier, if an exercise hurts you for whatever reason, find another exercise alternative that doesn't. Now, the sensation associated with muscle fatigue or feeling the burn isn't what we're talking about here. We're talking about aches and pains that exist outside the gym or flare up when you perform certain movements.

These problems may need time to heal through rest, or they may simply be injuries, which are compromised areas of your body that can no longer tolerate the high load and do not improve. Either way you're not helping the situation by training through pain. In fact, you very well could be making things worse and causing further damage, which could take a painful area from something you can train through to something that's debilitating. That said, it's always a good idea to have a qualified medical professional assess any aches and pains rather than trying to play doctor yourself.

Additionally, there are many exercise options in this book for you to choose from. If a certain upper-body pushing exercise hurts you, for example, simply experiment with the other upper-body pushing options until you find one that you can do without pain.

Another option to help you work around painful areas is to simply limit the range of motion of the exercise. Let's say that you can perform a squat exercise without pain, but when you get near the bottom of the squat, the pain starts. In cases like this, simply reduce the range of motion and only go as low as you can without creating pain.

All training (i.e., exercise) is an applied stress to the body. It is this stress that causes the body to adapt by becoming stronger, bigger, and fitter in order to accommodate the stress with more efficiency and to better tolerate it to reduce the chance of injury. That said, smart training is about applying enough stress to our body to make it adapt without applying too much stress and overloading the tissues to the point where they become damaged. When there is pain, your tolerance to stress becomes severely reduced and you're much more likely to create distress (instead of stress), which, again, is likely to make things worse. The goal is to fit the exercises in this book to you (how you move and what feels right to you), not to try to fit yourself to the moves in this book.

Take Time Off From Training

This is another point that should be common sense, but many people don't do it, so it's worth briefly covering. Every few months of using the training programs in this book, you should take off several days from your workouts to allow your body and mind to recover and refocus. Taking a rest break of 4 to 7 days every 8 to 12 weeks or so can be a valuable method of avoiding overtraining, and it can also get you hungry to get back into the gym, which can help you avoid getting in the habit of simply going through the motions.

Just because you're taking a break from the workouts in this book doesn't mean you have to do nothing at all. During your days off, try to do some low-impact activities such as going for long walks, hikes, bike rides, or swims. Also, yoga can be a great option for your active rest periods. If you're already doing yoga each week, as recommended earlier, you can simply increase your yoga practice in your deloading (rest) week.

Additionally, you don't have to use metabolic strength training methods for all of your training programs throughout the year. In fact, when fat loss is your primary training goal, I recommend you use two of the four-week metabolic strength training programs provided in this book—that's 2-months of training. And, then do 4-6 weeks of traditional-style strength training to focus on your strength. Doing this not only keeps things fresh, but it also ensures that your body doesn't become overly adapted to one particular style of training. Plus, taking 4-6 weeks to focus on improving your strength can only help you get more out of your metabolic strength training workouts when you go back to them because you'll be able to perform the exercises with better control and with a higher intensity.

The beauty of the metabolic strength training system is its versatility and simplicity. By using the tools you've learned in this chapter and throughout the book, you will safely and effectively get into record shape. Although I've provided a wide variety of exercises and protocols that you can use regardless of equipment or training environment, I encourage you to use the methods in this book as inspiration to develop your own metabolic strength training complexes, combinations, and circuits and workout programs using these methods.

This book is a powerful fat-loss weapon that is now locked and loaded in your training arsenal. All you've got to do is use it!

References

CHAPTER 1

1. Migliaccio S, Greco EA, et al. Skeletal alterations in women affected by obesity. Aging Clin Exp Res. 2013 Sep 24.
2. Ackerman IN, Osborne RH. Obesity and increased burden of hip and knee joint disease in Australia: results from a national survey. BMC Musculoskelet Disord. 2012 Dec 20;13:254
3. Sundquist K, Winkleby M, Li X, Ji J, Hemminki K, Sundquist J. Title: Familiar transmission of coronary heart disease: A cohort study of 80,214 Swedish adoptees linked to their biological and adoptive parents. Am Heart J. 2011 Aug;162(2):317-23.
4. Michael Craig Miller M.D. Understanding Depression. Harvard Medical School. March 1, 2011
5. Schoenfeld TJ, Rada P, et al. Physical exercise prevents stress-induced activation of granule neurons and enhances local inhibitory mechanisms in the dentate gyrus. J Neurosci. 2013 May 1;33(18):7770-7.
6. Driver HS, Taylor SR. Exercise and sleep. Sleep Med Rev. 2000 Aug;4(4):387-402.

CHAPTER 2

1. Brad Schoenfled. The MAX Muscle Plan. Human Kinetics Publishing. 2013. Pg.206
2. George Abboud, et. al., "Effects of Load-Volume on EPOC After Acute Bouts of Resistance Training in Resistance-Trained Men," Journal of Strength and Conditioning Research, 27(7), 2013.
3. Chantal A. Vella, PhD, Len Kravitz, PhD. Exercise After-Burn: A Research Update. IDEA Fitness Journal. November 2004.
4. Willis et al., J App Phys., vol. 113 no. 12: 1831-1837; 2012.
5. Heden T, Lox C, Rose P, Reid S, Kirk EP. One-set resistance training elevates energy expenditure for 72 h similar to three sets. Eur J Appl Physiol. 2011 Mar;111(3):477-84.
6. Bahr R, Sejersted OM. 1991. Effect of intensity of exercise on excess postexercise oxygen consumption. *Metabolism, 40(8), 836-841.*
7. Phelain JF, et al. 1997. Postexericse energy expenditure and substrate oxidation in young women resulting from exercise bouts of different intensity. *Journal of the American College of Nutrition,* 16(2), 140-146.
8. Yingling VR, Yack HJ, and White SC. 1996. The Effect of Rearfoot Motion on Attenuation of the Impulse Wave at Impact During Running. *Journal of Applied Biomechanics.* (Champaign, IL: Human Kinetics), 12, 313-325.

CHAPTER 3

1. Frank M. Sacks, M.D., George A. Bray, M.D., et al. Comparison of Weight-Loss Diets with Different Compositions of Fat, Protein, and Carbohydrates. N Engl J Med 2009; 360:859-873February 26, 2009
2. Zalesin KC, Franklin BA, Lillystone MA, et al. Differential loss of fat and lean mass in the morbidly obese after bariatric surgery. Metab Syndr Relat Disord. 2010;8(1):15–20. doi:10.1089/met.2009.0012.
3. Santarpia L, Contaldo F, Pasanisi F. Body composition changes after weight-loss interventions for overweight and obesity. Clin Nutr. 2013;32(2):157–161. doi:10.1016/j.clnu.2012.08.016.
4. Chaston TB, Dixon JB, O'Brien PE. Changes in fat-free mass during significant weight loss: a systematic review. International Journal of Obesity (2005). 2007;31(5):743–750.
5. Redman LM, Heilbronn LK, Martin CK, et al. Metabolic and Behavioral Compensations in Response to Caloric Restriction: Implications for the Maintenance of Weight Loss. PLoS One. 2009;4(2):e4377 EP –. doi:doi:10.1371/journal.pone.0004377.
6. Garthe I, Raastad T, Refsnes PE, Koivisto A, Sundgot-Borgen J. Effect of two different weight-loss rates on body composition and strength and power-related performance in elite athletes. Int J Sport Nutr Exerc Metab. 2011;21(2):97–104.
7. Mero AA, Huovinen H, Matintupa O, et al. Moderate energy restriction with high protein diet results in healthier outcome in women. J Int Soc Sports Nutr. 2010;7(1):4. doi:10.1186/1550-2783-7-4.
8. Martin CK, Das SK, Lindblad L, et al. Effect of calorie restriction on the free-living physical activity levels of nonobese humans: results of three randomized trials. J Appl Physiol. 2011;110(4):956–963. doi:10.1152/japplphysiol.00846.2009.

9. Mozaffarian D, Katan M, Ascherio A, Stampfer M, Willett W. Trans fatty acids and cardiovascular disease. N Engl J Med. 2006;354:1601-13.

10. Amanda R. Kirpitch, MA, RD, CDE, LDN and Melinda D. Maryniuk, MEd, RD, CDE, LDN. The 3 R's of Glycemic Index: Recommendations, Research, and the Real World. Clinical Diabetes October 2011 vol. 29 no. 4 155-159

11. Hall KD. What is the required energy deficit per unit weight loss? International Journal of Obesity (2005). 2008;32(3):573–576. doi:10.1038/sj.ijo.0803720.

12. van der Ploeg GE, Brooks AG, Withers RT, Dollman J, Leaney F, Chatterton BE. Body composition changes in female bodybuilders during preparation for competition. Eur J Clin Nutr. 2001;55(4):268–277. doi:10.1038/sj.ejcn.1601154.

13. Withers RT, Noell CJ, Whittingham NO, Chatterton BE, Schultz CG, Keeves JP. Body composition changes in elite male bodybuilders during preparation for competition. Aust J Sci Med Sport. 1997;29(1):11–16. Available at: http://www.ncbi.nlm.nih.gov/pubmed/9127683.

14. Erica R Goldstein, Tim Ziegenfuss, et al. International society of sports nutrition position stand: caffeine and performance. Journal of the International Society of Sports Nutrition 2010, 7:5

15. Holmstrup, ME, Owns CM, Fairchild TJ, Kanaley JA. Effect of meal frequency on glucose and insulin excursions over the course of a day. *The European e-Journal of Clinical Nutrition and Metabolism.* Volume 5, Issue 6, e277-e280. December 2010.

16. Halton T, Hu F. 2004. The effects of high protein diets on thermogenesis, satiety, and weight loss: A critical review. *Journal of the American College of Nutrition.* Volume 23, 373-385.

CHAPTER 9

1. Medeiros HS Jr, Mello RS, et al. Planned intensity reduction to maintain repetitions within recommended hypertrophy range. Int J Sports Physiol Perform. 2013 Jul;8(4):384-90. Epub 2012 Nov 19.

CHAPTER 10

1. Sale DG. Neural adaptation to resistance training. Med Sci Sports Exerc. 1988 Oct;20(5 Suppl):S135-45.

2. DeFreitas JM, Beck TW, et al. An examination of the time course of training-induced skeletal muscle hypertrophy. Eur J Appl Physiol. 2011 Nov;111(11):2785-90.

3. Seynnes OR, de Boer M, Narici MV. Early skeletal muscle hypertrophy and architectural changes in response to high-intensity resistance training. J Appl Physiol (1985). 2007 Jan;102(1):368-73.

4. Folland JP, Williams AG. The adaptations to strength training : morphological and neurological contributions to increased strength. Sports Med. 2007;37(2):145-68.

About the Author

Coach Nick Tumminello is the owner of Performance University International, which provides hybrid strength training and conditioning for athletes and professional educational programs for trainers and coaches all over the world.

As an educator, Coach Nick has become known as the Trainer of Trainers. He has presented at international fitness conferences in Iceland, China, and Canada. He has been a featured presenter at conferences held by such organizations as IDEA, NSCA, DCAC, and ECA, along with teaching staff trainings at fitness clubs throughout the United States. Nick holds workshops and mentorship programs in his hometown of Fort Lauderdale, Florida. He has produced more than 15 instructional DVDs and is a CEC provider for ACE and NASM.

Nick has been a fitness professional since 1998 and co-owned a private training center in Baltimore, Maryland, from 2001 to 2011. He has worked with a variety of exercise enthusiasts of all ages and fitness levels, including physique and performance athletes from the amateur to the professional ranks. From 2002 to 2011, Nick served as the strength and conditioning coach for the Ground Control MMA fight team and as is a consultant and expert for clothing and equipment companies such as Sorinex, Dynamax, Hylete, and Reebok.

Nick's articles have appeared in over 30 major health and fitness magazines, including Men's Health, Men's Fitness, Oxygen, Muscle Mag, Fitness RX, Sweat RX, Status, Train Hard

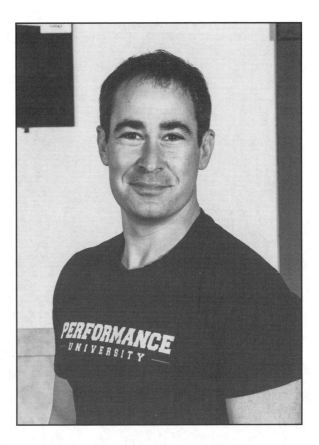

Fight Easy, Fighters Only, and Fight! Nick is also a featured contributor to several popular fitness training websites. He has been featured in two New York Times best-selling exercise books, on the front page of Yahoo.com and Youtube.com, and in the ACE Personal Trainer Manual, Fourth Edition.

Nick writes a popular fitness training blog at PerformanceU.net.

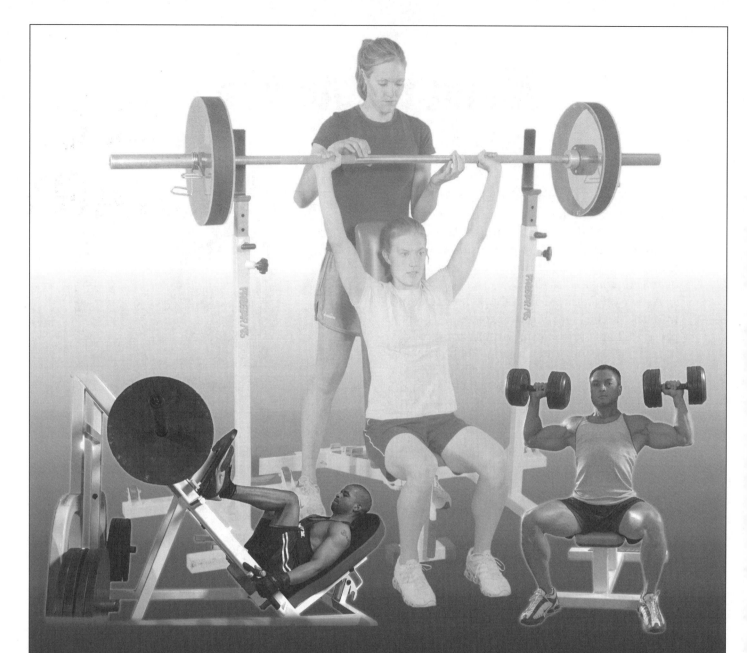
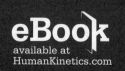